HAIRLOOM

A Woman's Generational Guide to
Hair Care, Wholeness & Balance for Life

Angie Allen

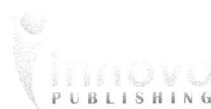

innovo
PUBLISHING

Published by Innovo Publishing, LLC
www.innovopublishing.com
1-888-546-2111

innovo
PUBLISHING

Providing Full-Service Publishing Services for Christian Authors, Artists & Ministries:
Books, eBooks, Audiobooks, Music, Film & Courses

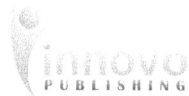

HAIRLOOM
A Woman's Generational Guide to Hair Care, Wholeness & Balance for Life

All scripture is taken from the King James Version (KJV) of the Bible.

Library of Congress Control Number: 2019908582
ISBN: 978-1-61314-505-0

Cover Design & Interior Layout: Innovo Publishing, LLC

Printed in the United States of America
U.S. Printing History
First Edition: 2020

Acknowledgments

I must begin with all glory, honor, and praise to my Lord and Savior Jesus Christ for allowing me to be chosen to conceive and birth this ministry.

To my husband, for his personal sacrificial investment and support for this opportunity: your determination and drive in ministry inspires me to live with no regrets.

Due to witnessing undesirable challenges that my mom faced as a cosmetologist, I originally rejected the entire hair care industry. I am grateful for her perseverance through pain, two knee surgeries, discomfort, disappointment, and the challenge of serving women for thirty years. She taught me how to keep business and personal matters separate while making others feel special and appreciated.

To my dad, for his insightful talks and always encouraging me to go the second mile.

To all of the clientele that has supported me through many transitions in ministry, time constraints, and location movement, and who has expressed autonomy of their hair care needs: I appreciate you for embracing the vision of not only *having* a healthy head of hair but also *investing* in your own head of hair.

Contents

Journal Introduction & Preparation

An *heirloom* is perhaps an antique or some kind of jewelry that has been passed down for generations through family members. Beliefs, ideologies, and practices can also be considered heirlooms, as they are passed down from one generation to the next and can affect one's identity, confidence, and self-esteem. An heirloom could be something as simple as a broach or ink pen, but what matters most is the significance and events surrounding that object. What was transpiring in that person's life, how valuable that object was in the whole scheme of economics, and the purpose and importance of the item to its original owner is what makes the heirloom important.

While considering the *why* for this journal, I could think of several reasons to abort the mission because of the need for more important priorities and aspirations in life. However, as I considered the past and how important my hair has been in my life, I had to press through the doubts and fears of releasing this opportunity. Just as an heirloom is something important enough to keep and considered valuable enough to pass down to the next generation, our health and wellness practices have just as much merit. Through my nursing and trichological studies, I discovered that health history has a major effect on future decisions.

So why did I name this journal *Hairloom*? I have studied the hair industry and its clientele for almost three decades and have noticed that we tend to receive and apply things that are passed down from our forefathers. Many people trust medical practitioners with their general health and wellness decisions without giving it a second thought. However, every part of our body's purpose is extremely important and should be understood. Hair has a purpose, and although it may not be a priority, it could become extremely inconvenient to have had something and lose it due to a lack of knowledge.

Therefore, I decided to create an opportunity in the form of a journal to serve as an heirloom to be passed down from one generation to the next. I have seen heirloom books and journals that tell the story of a loved one that helps to inform, educate, and inspire one to face challenges, and offers a blueprint of possible ways to address personal questions about one's insecurities or idiosyncrasies. Some heirlooms serve as a foundation from which to build and create a mindset to strive for more. Either way, a heads up about one's self can provide much-needed insight and encouragement to move past challenges with proactive knowledge and solutions.

My desire is to create an opportunity for you to not only share your own hair journey but also get to know more about yourself and simultaneously empower the next generation. Ultimately, I want you to see how important every part of your existence is to someone else. Yes, even your hair. Hair tells a lot about how we view ourselves, how we take care of ourselves, and the influence others have in our lives.

I would like to begin by sharing a little of my "journeymony" with you. For years, I complained about my hair and how fine the texture is. People would always say, "You got that good hair." Well, I didn't think it was good because my hair was not thick enough to hold the latest styles. It would grow as long as I desired, but year after year, I found myself dissatisfied with it. I would look at other people's hair, especially the thicker hair, and desire just a little more density in the crown of my head. It didn't help that my forehead was a little more prominent than I desired, with not enough density to cover it and still have volume throughout the rest of my style. For years I cut it in layers to give the appearance of volume and density that really was not there. The slightest bit of oil applied would weigh down any style I tried to achieve to a flat wrap. There seemed to be no hope until I began studying in the field of trichology and gained knowledge that had not been taught in cosmetology school. It was there that I finally began to become more confident and grateful for my hair.

The results were amazing, as I began to apply the same information that I share in this journal. First, my hair grew to a length that I had never had in my entire life. Second, the elasticity of my hair was strengthened, and I could use products that did not make me look like a wet cat by the head. Third, I learned how to properly handle my hair instead of trying to bully and manipulate it into what I wanted it to do. More importantly, I began to see results in my clients that decided to embrace the challenge. Those that began the journey with me over seven years ago have overcome different hair and scalp challenges and are more confident in their hair care practices. Believe it or not, some of them only schedule appointments for their chemical services and are still able to maintain the length and proper care of their hair. Therefore, it's not all about regular visits to the salon. It only requires knowledge, patience, and application. Anyone can experience a change in the health of their hair and scalp with a few minor adjustments.

If you are anything like me, I like to read, but I don't prefer a lot of fluff to make a book longer than what it needs to be to get to the point. Therefore, I have purposely made this a small, "quick guide" to give you enough info to get you started on your journey to more *manageable*, *viable*, and *protected*—what I will call *MVP*—hair. Also, I have created my own hair terminology throughout this journal. Words like *hairadigm shift*, *hairginity*, and *pro-hairbition*, just to name few, will hopefully keep you engaged and cause new neurocircuitry to fire as you are introduced to these concepts. Please be advised that all situations and circumstances are different, and depending on the present condition of your hair, some extra adjustments or consultations may be required. Either way, you will notice a difference, and others will also.

With life and all of the possibilities of setbacks and challenges, hair probably places next to last in the whole scheme of your priority list; but I believe that you desire to make changes because you picked up this journal. Changes will be necessary—maybe more for some than others; but either way, you will get results based on your effort.

ACCOUNTABILITY

If you are taking this journey alone, I would suggest that you reconsider, because I have found that accountability is important and very helpful in difficult times. I will never forget when I had a new client that I was a little reluctant to accept help. At that time, I was very selective of my clientele because I needed people that were willing to follow instructions in order to have full autonomy to produce what I knew was achievable. At this time, I did not consider their health issues or previous practices; I just wanted them to make adjustments based on my recommendations, and over time, I realized the importance of the things that I share in this journal to preface the journey.

This client—that I will refer to as VIP—was over fifty years of age, never had hair longer than above her shoulder, and her hair appeared to be thinning due to breakage in the crown. Unfortunately, she was not interested in wearing a wig while recovering, but she did agree to a big chop that only left two rotations on a size blue roller to set her over processed strands. I remember instructing her to avoid sleeping or laying on rollers—period. One day, she decided to be a little lazy and laid down to take a quick nap. She said that her husband told her, "Now didn't she tell you not to lay on rollers? If you are going to invest in your hair care, you have to obey the rules." *Wow!* I wanted to have a celebration party just for him holding her accountable for what she told him she needed to do. These are the kinds of people you need in your ear during this journey.

Of course, this journal only has capacity for one year. If used properly, it should only take one year for you to see your discipline, or lack thereof, concerning your hair/scalp care. During this time, this journal will help you learn about your body and your general wellness while challenging you to look at each strand of hair as an opportunity to grow and develop in your personal life.

Indulge me, as I paint a picture to parallel your hair and your life. Your head or scalp represents your life or foundation for living, while each strand—and there are thousands of them—represents opportunities, events, relationships, and challenges. Depending on the area of the head, the strands have more or less access to your attention. (I hope this is not too deep, but I want to express the importance of every part of our anatomy and its significance in life.) My spiritual leader says, "First natural, then spiritual," and I believe that our natural hair has spiritual significance and gives insight into areas of our lives that we may not readily see without some introspection. Our desires, habits, thoughts, and choices are influenced by things around us and should not be haphazardly considered. So, ask someone that you know cares about your entire life to hold you accountable during this *hairloom* journey.

The thing I like the most about hair is its preprogrammed ability to grow every day, yielding a minimum of six inches per year, depending on your DNA. Some journeys are direct and focused, while others may experience distractions and detours along the way. However, with a clear vision, guide, and path, you could see progress and have positive reinforcement opportunity within the first year of your journey. As you may have noticed by now, this is much deeper than just taking care of your hair and scalp. This journey will result in a new way of taking care of *you*, while potentially inspiring future generations.

VISION

Without a vision, your hair will perish.

To stay focused, you will write your vision for your hair (found at the end of this introduction). This vision should be placed in areas where you handle your hair on a regular basis. Also, I recommend that you memorize it in the event that you are away from your vision document. Share your vision with your accountability partner, and ask them to remind you and encourage you weekly to stay the course. This opportunity for change can also spill over into other areas of your life, like the events, relationships, challenges, and opportunities that each strand represents in your life. Here is the first vision I spoke for a couple of years over my hair and scalp:

> *My hair increases in density and thickness every day*
> *My hair is growing longer, stronger, healthier, more manageable, more elastic, and shinier*
> *My scalp and follicular activity are in optimal health and properly function to produce healthy hair*
> *I have no breakage or premature shedding*
> *My hair is my glory, and I give God all the glory in Jesus's name*

I noticed that my vision carried me through the more challenging times of my journey. Since my hair is long, it's a little harder to cut more than a few inches at a time. However, I still had some old color-treated and relaxed strands that were causing some tangling issues during my hair care regimen. (I would like to introduce you to my terminology that I will use to represent hair care regimen: *hairgistics*—I will discuss more on this later.) This frustrated me, and I eventually stopped wearing my hair at all. During the winter months, I could cover it with a turban and caps because of the weather. This helped so I wouldn't have to handle it as much in its fragile state, but it also created an environment for me to be lazy and skip deep conditioning. It wasn't too long before I figured out that this was a critical part of my *hairgistics*.

Just as there are different seasons of the year, we also experience different seasons in life. We have to respect the process and understand that regardless of our greatest intentions, we will still experience a gamut of opportunities that cause our schedules and plans to be adjusted. This is why *Hairloom* is a great way to see your life unfold and reveal patterns and cycles that need to be addressed and possibly eliminated.

I noticed a pattern in my life and my clientele that called for a change in hair color or style—where one would feel out of control or trapped in situations or relationships without hope for immediate change. These times could come in the form of relationships in marriage, family, on the job, school, or internal issues that have not been expressed. Either way, what is going on internally will eventually manifest, and unfortunately, haircare is one of the first things to be reprioritized.

Speaking of prioritizing, I remember when salon visits made every two weeks was a big deal, and one expected for all of the hair challenges to be overcome within that one visit with no personal midweek responsibility required. Well, we have seen a shift in the hair industry over the last decade, from needing cosmetologists to needing hair seamstresses, dermatologists, and trichologists because *hairgistics* have become obsolete; meanwhile all the blame is placed on the stylist and chemical damage.

PRIORITY

Based on your vision, your *hairgistics* must become your priority in order to reach your goal. If your vision is as simple as *discontinue using heated tools*, this journal is not for you. However, if you would like to experience the growth of MVP hair/scalp with length retention of at least six inches, then a certain environment has to be created to support this vision.

Prioritizing your hair care needs requires strategic decisions, and this is where we have to be intentional but also realistic. I am sure that most would like to handle this journey alone, but that may not be feasible with your schedule or limited knowledge of how hair works. While others may desire to continue visiting the salon that is most comfortable—and this too could pose a challenge because some stylists are not able, willing, or knowledgeable about how trichology works.

Trichology is a branch of dermatology that studies the anatomy, physiology, and pathology of the hair and the epidermis (scalp). Its priority is health over style, and herein lies the issue for stylists or traditional cosmetologists. They are trained and proficient in making you look and feel good about yourself when you get out of the chair. On the other hand, a trichologist may have to have a counseling session to reinforce the importance of why certain decisions have to be made to achieve desired results. In other words, you may not be in a position to wear a style while being treated.

For example, if you break a limb, it will need a cast. If the hair is broken, it needs reinforcement and protection to eliminate further damage. There is no way to continue to do the same thing to your hair and get different results. The last thing your doctor is concerned with is how that cast or ankle boot is going to look with your Sunday outfit. Therefore, let's decide now if we are going to do it alone or find someone that will be willing to follow your *hairgistics* during your *hairloom*.

The responsibility will be the same, except on one hand, you will be totally responsible for everything, and on the other hand, you will have someone else to share in the responsibility. Either way, you will have to learn how to do it all and teach your stylist how to do it for you. My desire is to teach a generation of people to understand and at least know how to do their own hair, if necessary.

I believe God created the abundance of hair to allow for trial and error opportunities. Think about it: every other part of our body that we have immediate access to only has two members apiece—two legs, two arms, two hands (extra fingers = more prone to injury), two eyes, two ears, etc. I believe He gave us more strands of hair because He wanted us to enjoy it and learn about it at our convenience.

In order to have a healthy scalp and hair environment, you will need to apply *hairgistics*—hair logistics—for your particular needs. Therefore, we will need a coordinated set of products and techniques to address your particular needs. It will include shampoo, conditioner, moisture, and oil. Most fail to understand that what is done in secret will be rewarded openly. It's unfortunate that most people believe that having their hair done when the style no longer looks presentable is sufficient and responsible.

Some believe that although the rest of the body requires daily cleansing, shampooing is only needed if the head begins to itch too much. This is very disconcerting and needs to be rejected once and for all.

Think about it: hair extends from the same body that all the rest of your body parts extend from, whether it's an arm or leg or unmentionable hairs in other places; scalp hair is still attached to the same foundation or body. If you already have to shower or bathe more than once in a day during summer months, whatever you were doing to produce the sweat and odor has also happened while your hair was attached to your head.

Heat is heat, sweat is sweat, and stink is stink. Furthermore, you know you have smelled your hair at some point; whether it was while you were in the shower or in the shampoo bowl, you smelled something that was emitted off of your head. Even if it doesn't itch; I don't care if its braided, under a wig, or slicked back with plenty of sweet-smelling products, it's still dirty if you didn't shampoo.

In a perfect world, shampooing would be a daily event, and all would be decent and in order; however, there is also something called *having a style and looking presentable with little to no effort* that is coveted. Herein lies the challenge and where compromise and responsible decisions are needed. At the very least, once a week is acceptable. If you are more active and sweat more or work out, shampooing no less than every three days is acceptable. Either way, any time after seven days is unacceptable. Equally important is the responsibility of deep conditioning after each shampoo and applying a leave-in conditioner when deep conditioning is not processed. Shampooing and conditioning is only the foundation and still requires support products that help to maintain the viability of healthy hair. Moisture and oil applied after the hair has been styled helps to maintain hydration and shine until next *hairgistics* is performed.

Here are some tips to follow that are required for a successful hair journey:

1. Document your vision.

2. Share with your accountability partner.

3. Based on your time chart, find time for the next year to dedicate to this journey.

4. Decide if you are going to take the challenge or allow your stylist/trichologist to assist you.

5. Purchase products/supplies.

6. Watch tutorial videos.

7. Speak your vision every time you touch your hair or look in the mirror (*memorize it*). It is seed for the growth that you are about to experience.

8. Follow the weekly journal entries thoroughly; your generations are depending on you.

9. Even if you fall behind, it doesn't matter; just keep up with your dates and pictures to document your progress.

10. Pay attention to patterns that cause detours along your journey.

11. Reinforce your goals with your accountability partner, and don't give up.

12. Post your progress pictures in a conspicuous place to encourage yourself in the busy and tough times.

RESPONSIBILITY

So far we have *accountability*, *vision*, and *priority*. Next is *responsibility*—how to create a journal that will serve as an *hairloom* for the next generation. Sometimes our goals and aspirations have to be greater than just about oneself. When you know that someone else is depending on your guidance and experience, you tend to take the opportunity a little more seriously. Whether you believe it or not, you have already begun passing down all types of information to the next generation, spoken and unspoken.

For example, I remember when my five-year-old cousin decided to cut her bangs. Unfortunately, she cut them almost to the scalp, and when her mother asked her why she did it, she said, "Well, Auntie said that when you cut the hair it will grow back longer." Little did she know, Auntie was not talking about cutting hair just for the purpose of growing more; it was to trim the ends that were split and causing breakage. I am not sure if her Auntie explained the entire process of trimming damaged hair, but my cousin figured that she had enough info and was ready to apply the knowledge without further instruction. Needless to say, it took a little while for her bangs to grow back, and my aunt made sure that she let her wear them just like they were cut. Hilarious!

We must have the whole story to successfully take care of our health. That's why we need a guide or road map to follow in order to avoid unforeseen obstacles that could detour us from desired results. Although the hair is growing a little every day, in a year, you should expect six inches. But if you are having to trim an inch every month after a relaxer, you will not see an increase in length unless your hair is color treated and you can watch your color move farther and farther away from the roots.

Let's begin with a fun pop quiz of prior knowledge and hair care techniques to determine if the current logic should be continued or discarded.

Pop Quiz

1. The foundation for a healthy head of hair is to keep the ends trimmed.

   True   **False**

2. All shampoos serve the same purpose, which is to clean the hair and scalp.

   True   **False**

3. Proper conditioning is very important because it helps to repair hair that becomes damaged, thin, and broken.

   True   **False**

4. Brushing can scratch your scalp and tear your hair.

   True   **False**

5. The most effective way to remove tangles is by holding the hair at the root and raking through the ends until tangles have been released.

   True   **False**

6. Shampooing is required when your style does not look presentable.

   True   **False**

7. The number one cause of hair breakage is using super strength relaxers.

   True   **False**

8. Dandruff is an indication that hair is growing.

   True   **False**

9. A sensitive scalp is a damaged scalp.

   True   **False**

10. The safest styling technique is a roller set.

    True   **False**

I have provided the answers at the back of the journal (appendix) so you won't be tempted to cheat. Yes, some of the questions are tricky, but I want you to see how uneducated the population has been concerning hair and scalp care. I remember a time when the scalp was not even mentioned in matters of the hair. Focusing solely on the hair and ignoring the scalp is like going to a dermatologist and asking for a consultation to get a hairpiece.

Another part of your responsibility is to answer a questionnaire to assess your present situation. Just as any map app needs your current location to navigate the final destination, we must begin with where you are now and make adjustments to move to the desired place. Here are a few things to consider that may affect your hair: *hairgistics*, new *hairtrition*, exercise, your *hairadigm*, and schedule organization, just to name a few. We will chart these practices to get an idea of the adjustments that need to be made or continued to create a proper environment for health and wellness, not just for your hair but for the entire body. They are a package deal, and by now, you have probably noticed some patterns in your life that have a direct correlation to unwanted changes in your health and hair.

Questionnaire: Where are you now?

Allergies? Yes _____ No _____

Medications: _____

_____

History of balding in your family? Yes _____ No _____

Who: _____

History of scalp problems in your family? Yes _____ No _____

Type: _____

Who: _____

Do you wear a chemical? Yes _____ No _____

Type: _____

When was your last Chemical? _____

How often? _____ At Salon: _____ At home: _____

When chemicals are being applied, does your scalp: Itch _____ Tingle _____ Burn _____

Do you use any semi-permanent or temporary colors? Yes _____ No _____

What type? _____

Where is your hair shampooed? Home _____ Salon _____ Both _____

Name hair products you use the most: Shampoo _____ Conditioner _____

Styling or support products: _____

"Product Junkie" tendency: _____

Do you use heated tools on your hair? Yes _____ No _____

How often? _____

Type? _____

What type of pillowcase do you sleep on? Satin _____ Cotton _____ Other _____

How do you dress your hair for bed? _____

What hair products do you use every day? _____

Scalp

Does your scalp itch? Yes _____ No _____

Does your scalp flake? Yes _____ No _____

Are there any tender areas? Yes _____ No _____

Hair

Is there any breakage? Yes _____ No _____

Is there any dryness? Yes _____ No _____

Are there any thinning areas? Yes _____ No _____ Location: _____

Do your meals include: Breakfast _____ Lunch _____ Dinner _____

How are meals prepared: Home _____ Fast food _____ Restaurants _____

Hairloom

Daily water intake: _____

Vitamins/Supplements: _____

Consistent use _____ Not consistent _____

Exercise _____ Sedentary lifestyle _____

Married _____ Single _____ With children _____ Without children _____

Age _____

Career _____ School _____ Job _____ Ministry _____ Traveler _____ Entrepreneur _____

I have provided a miniature daily time chart so you can see if you have time to take on this opportunity. Hopefully this will provide a brief overlook of what your schedule looks like. You should only provide what is consistently done every week on a regular basis. For example, if you attend service on Sundays, chart that. If you work a 9–5, chart that. If you have an exercise class on Thursdays, chart that. Whatever you do every week that cannot be changed or adjusted, be sure to record that information in the chart provided.

Time	Sun	Mon	Tues	Wed	Thurs	Fri	Sat
4am							
5am							
6am							
7am							
8am							
9am							
10am							
11am							
12pm							
1pm							
2pm							
3pm							
4pm							
5pm							
6pm							
7pm							
8pm							
9pm							
10pm–4am							

JOURNEMONY TIME

The following is an example of what you can write for your first entry in the "Journemony" section of this journal:

My *hairloom*:

Mom's side: Two generations of hair stylists or what were called beauticians. (1) Mom: medium texture hair; able to grow and maintain thirty-plus inches in length after sixty-six years of age; general health issues and several surgeries due to stress and wear and tear of the body. My mom and I have the most length, at least below the bra strap, of all of our family members on both sides. This indicates that there was a breach in how to take care of the hair that was passed down through our generations. (2) Grandmother: eighty-four years of age; no surgeries or hospitalizations other than childbirth; hair short to ear length until she allowed me to start taking care of it seven years ago.

Dad's side: No hair experience. (1) My father is the only male in the family with density issues in the crown; general health issues corrected by adjusting diet and exercise. (2) Grandmother turned one hundred years old as of 2018; no surgeries other than childbirth; reasonable health; excellent memory to date; fine, short hair throughout life.

My hair journey: Since 2007, I have been able to maintain at least twenty-four inches of hair while transitioning from a chemical relaxer and color and trimming quarterly. Three years ago, my density was challenged, and I noticed thinning after the chemical and heat processes due to *hairgistic* issues. Thankfully, I am in recovery and doing much better. As soon as this journal is released, I will be cutting the remaining chemically treated strands that I have nurtured for the purpose of this journey.

HAIRADIGM

My spiritual leader says that there are many voices and none without significance. This means that every word, yours and others, has a meaning and a message, and whether you believe it or not, it affects how you think, feel, and respond. Imagine a house with columns that support the front porch. If you were to remove those columns, they would have to be replaced with more columns to continue to support the structure of that house. Therefore, a *hairadigm* is your present columns that support how you view your hair; but a *hairadigm shift* is the new columns that this journal will provide for you to replace the old perspective, knowledge, and experience you have encountered.

I can remember becoming very insecure about how I looked at a young age. An authority figure in my life told my mom that I needed bangs because my forehead was more pronounced than they thought it should have been for me to look pretty. Well, I found myself not even wanting to go to the mailbox or be in the presence of anyone without my bangs until after marriage. I know, this is so sad because bangs or not, I should have never picked up that insecurity. Whether it was true or not—and I believed it to be true—I should have known that my forehead did not define me or take away from the potential that was on the inside of me to be the best human that I could be. Hence, *hairadigm* to *hairadigm shift*.

Although this part is very personal, I want you to be totally honest concerning these questions because one day, your great-granddaughter may pick this journal up and see that she is experiencing some of the same challenges concerning her appearance as you have. However, by the end of this journal, she will come to resolve, through your words of encouragement, to appreciate her qualities, characteristics, and *hairginity* (another term I prefer to use that represents hair that is void of chemical, heat, and mechanical manipulation) that make her unique. Her introspection via this *hairloom* will allow her to face her own issues and release any attachments that could develop into insecurities.

I will never forget a young lady that decided to "go natural." (By the way, there is no such thing as "going natural"; you will forever grow your natural hair from the scalp. It never leaves, unless you go bald.) This young lady finally grew enough hair to feel comfortable enough to cut the remaining chemically processed hair off of the ends. However, because her grandmother had such influence in her life, she never reclaimed her *hairginity* because it "didn't look professional or neat enough" for her grandmother's approval. So what did she do? She wore braids or used heat to straighten her hair, not realizing that all she was doing was over processing it with heat, and she could have just kept her relaxer to do that. To this day, all because of the influence and opinion of others, she has not been able to achieve MVP hair.

It's sad when we don't know our own worth and realize that we are made the way we are for a reason. What does your *hairadigm* sound like?

If you have ever declared or thought any of these statements, place a check in the box:

- ☐ My hair will never grow past a certain point.
- ☐ I wish my hair was longer, but it always breaks.
- ☐ My hair is too damaged to be helped.
- ☐ I don't have time to fool with my hair.
- ☐ It's more convenient to just wear a wig or extensions.
- ☐ I wish my hair was a different texture.
- ☐ Why does my hair have to be so "nappy"?
- ☐ I wish I could shave this stuff and just wear a bald fade.
- ☐ I would "go natural" but I wouldn't know what to do with it.
- ☐ My relaxers burn, but I can't live without them.
- ☐ I cannot wait past six weeks to relax my hair; it won't hold a style.
- ☐ I wish I had my other parents' hair than this mess.
- ☐ I am too old to try to grow some hair.
- ☐ I want to give my hair a break, but I need my color because of all this grey.
- ☐ I could never wear a wig; it's embarrassing.
- ☐ I feel more confident when I wear extensions.
- ☐ I look better with extensions.
- ☐ I seem to attract more positive attention when I wear extensions.
- ☐ Everybody else is wearing extensions; I am not going to get left behind.
- ☐ My hair is so damaged, I wish I could shave it and start over.
- ☐ Every time I experience a transition or challenge, I have to change my hair.
- ☐ My hair is all I have control over.
- ☐ If I wasn't natural, I would be able to be hired in more professional positions.
- ☐ I refuse to wear my natural hair to work because I could experience discrimination.

I am sure there are many more thoughts and conversations you have had about your hair that may not support what you truly desire. I desire that you prosper and be in health even as your soul prospers. I desire that everything about you be in the best condition that it can be. I desire that you get to a place where how you decide to wear your hair is because of preference and not because your hair is a problem. I believe that some of our challenges are presented because we have the solution inside of us to enhance someone else's journey.

Thank God for the inventor of the straightening comb—it served its time well, but I am sure it's because someone was trying to change the original appearance of the hair in the first place. But why? What was wrong with the hair, and what was it compared to? My spiritual leader says that comparing ourselves is not wise. I believe it's because there will always be something to be desired, and instead of focusing on what someone else has, we really should be trying to focus on the capacity that is already within.

If I covet your eighteen inches that fall right above the bra strap, I may never know that my hair really has capacity to hit the waistline. Who knows? One thing we can desire is optimum density, optimum length, and manageability, of which all creation has capacity. Texture and type are subjective and vary based on DNA. Yes, you can change it, but will it represent the best choice for your hair, health, and lifestyle?

Ultimately, I want this *hairloom* to be the motivator for you to become more knowledgeable about overall health and your *hairgistics*. This will not just be a one-year journey or a one-time *hairloom* to leave to your next generation; this is a lifelong guide to creating an environment for MVP (*manageable, viable,* and *protected)* hair/scalp and overall wellness.

In a few words, write a letter to the next generation that you believe would provide more insight into why you have chosen to pass down this *hairloom.*

_____
_____
_____
_____
_____
_____
_____
_____
_____
_____
_____

Whether your hair is natural or chemically altered, applying *hairgistics* is important because how your hair responds to style options can be greatly affected by product decisions. However, MVP hair/scalp can be produced by,
- making sure that you have a shampoo that cleans the scalp and strands
- using a conditioner that provides a protein and moisture balance
- properly applying and handling the strands, especially in their most fragile state while your hair is wet and dry
- applying support products between your *hairgistics* to keep the hair hydrated and manageable

GOAL AND VISION

- Grow at least six inches (God's allowance per person) with a healthy, uncompromised environment in the next year.
- Manipulate the hair as little as possible, and protect it with all your might.
- Keep hair clean conditioned, hydrated, and manageable at all times.

Remember, you are nurturing and watching something grow that's dead—a protein called keratin. Therefore, take the pressure off and realize that this is more about learning God's intention toward His creation than anything else. I will address this revelation at another time on another platform, because it is major and significant to salvation.

Now that we know where we are and where we desire to go, here is a quick map to reach your destination.

Five simple steps to remember each week: Section & Detangle, Shampoo, Condition, Protect

1. **Section** the hair in 4 to 6 sections, depending on your density.
2. **Detangle** each section by using your fingers to release any tangles or shed hair that may be causing hairs to congregate and create knots toward the ends of the hair.
3. **Shampoo** twice and rinse thoroughly each time.
4. **Condition** 15–30 minutes each week.
5. **Protect** your hair during manipulation while it is wet and dry by taking your time, using your fingers to detangle, and choosing styles and support products that will encourage MVP hair/scalp.

This *hairloom* is an excellent way to see growth and develop *hairgistics* for unforeseen challenges. Make note of how hair responds to products: itching, drying, shedding on the clothes, curl capacity, etc. Make note of seasonal changes that you notice with your hair and physiological challenges in your body.

HOW TO USE THE JOURNAL

Taking care of yourself is a personal investment. It will take time, but once you have created an environment for MVP hair, it will begin to work for you and reproduce a continual harvest. You will notice that I have divided the journal into different sections because I realize that some may not want to take a record of their entire life. Therefore, if you are somewhat comfortable with your schedule and don't foresee any issues with staying on track, by all means, just focus on the *Regimen, Journemory* and *Picture* portions of the journal, which will address all of the hair care education and help you create a successful *hairloom*.

Each month is divided into different categories or topics that are relevant to that particular time of the year. I tried to consider some of the issues that you may face with *hairgistics* during that particular time. Each week, I will focus on topics about how hair works from a trichological perspective while giving practical and applicable tips to support your journey. I love this system because it allows for strategic focus concerning *hairgistics* and tips from one week to the next. Even if you decided to skip the previous info, you can still be successful as you follow the week-by-week process of the journal. Also, no matter what month you begin, the topics, tips, and tutorials will guide you as well.

Since this journal is interactive, it will require your participation. Remember to envision yourself educating the next generation—your daughter, granddaughter, or maybe even great-granddaughter—about how to successfully take care of their hair by the practices, trials, and errors that you made.

This is not just about you; this is a very valuable and precious memory that you are preparing for someone you truly love and genuinely care about. Renounce all excuses and apply the instruction that this *hairloom* provides and this will serve as a new chapter. No matter where you start, you have already begun to make a difference just by taking the challenge to do something different. So congratulations on your first *hairloom*! And I pray that you experience health and wellness, not just for your hair but also for your mental, emotional, and physical well-being, which will transcend throughout your generations.

Goal

Each month you will write a goal. Your goals should support your vision statement to follow throughout the year. I recommend that you write it each month in your journal because it may change depending on your schedule and life in general.

The following is a list of topics that you will be charting throughout the *hairloom* as it relates to your stated goal. I desire for this to be multifunctional and to reveal a wide scope of your life, with details that will present patterns to learn about yourself. I will call them the 4 Rs:

1. Reflection
2. Responsibility
3. Regimen
4. Relaxation

Reflection

If you are like me, I prefer to decree my day by devoting time to build my spiritual perspective and reflect on God's will for my life. Therefore, I have provided a brief reflection each week for you to meditate on that will enhance your spiritual and emotional *hairloom*.

Responsibility

Each week you will be provided with a chart, like the following. In it, provide a snapshot of what you plan to do. Hopefully, this system will help to prioritize your life in order to experience a stress-free productive week that focuses not only on what needs to be done but also on strategically taking care of yourself.

Mon	
Tues	
Wed	
Thu	
Fri	
Sat	
Sun	

Record any extra scheduled tasks that could interfere with your normal routine. Taking thought for tomorrow is not recommended, so I recommend taking time each week to plan and prioritize your weekly schedule. This way, you can fully engage in the activities of your daily agenda.

I have found that *hairgistics* is normally one of the first things that is neglected when priorities change in your life. I believe that with a little planning, *hairgistics* should not have to suffer to attend to basic needs. If you follow the journal for at least three months, you will begin to see patterns that you may not have recognized. In my personal journal entries, I noticed that when life gets a little busy, I am faithful to journal for at least two weeks straight, and then I noticed that I would discontinue for about two weeks before I could get back on track. To avoid this inconsistency, I began to place my journal on my night stand, and it would be the first thing that I saw in the morning, causing me to pick it up and at least write something—just to stay on track. I have heard that it takes forty days to make or break a habit, so if nothing else is accomplished, try your very best to journal at least for forty days before getting off track. Sometimes you may have to record your info on your phone and go back and fill in the necessary info to avoid missing information that could later help you determine your patterns and procedures that work not only for your daily regimen but also your hair.

Regimen

Chart your *hairgistics*. *Hairgistics* is *hair logistics*, the detailed coordination, arrangement, or management of a complex operation that involves you, your stylist, your environment, and necessary tools to have a successful hair journey. By keeping record of your weekly *hairgistics*, you will be able to determine what combination of products, tools, and techniques create the desired results that you seek for MVP hair/scalp.

Each week you will fill out some information. Based on your results, you will be able to make adjustments if necessary and have a detailed record of the *hairgistics* that produced those results:

Shampoo (*yes or no; write product brands you are using*)

Conditioner (*yes or no; write product brands you are using*)

Leave-In (*yes or no; write product brands you are using*)

Support Product (*write the actual product brands you use*)

Conditioning time (*write the time you conditioned*)

Dryer Time (*write how long*) Air dry (*write how long*)

Protective Style (*write the type of protective style chosen*)

Detangle: Comb (*yes or no*) Finger (*yes or no*)

In the tables below, you will chart the observations made *before* you shampoo or begin your *hairgistics* for that week and *after* you have completed your *hairgistics*. Different products produce different results; therefore, it takes a few months to determine what *hairgistics* will work best for your hair. Since I cannot consult each person that takes the challenge, I cannot recommend what to use; so you will have to discover this part on your own. This is why I have provided so much detail of what to observe and chart, so you can make the best decision of what to use based on how your hair responds to the *hairgistics*. (The blank columns were provided to chart any other observations that I may not have included.)

Before

Dry	Shedding	Full		
Moist	Breaking	Frizzy		
Oily	Limp	Dull		
Stinky	Heavy	Itchy		
Tangled	Tight	Hard		

After

Dry	Shedding	Full		
Moist	Breaking	Frizzy		
Oily	Limp	Dull		
Stinky	Heavy	Itchy		
Tangled	Tight	Hard		

Make sure you have ample time for at least the first three months to become consistently acquainted with your hair and scalp needs to develop your *hairgistics*. To stay focused, refer to your vision and look at the visual picture of your goal.

Relaxation

In order to have balance, you must also schedule time to relax. I have provided some ideas of how to incorporate relaxation in your weekly schedule and ways to relieve stress that has become a normal part of your daily routine—even though you may not recognize it.

Journemony Time

I have also provided a space for you to encourage the next generation. Hopefully, you already have someone in mind that you would like to empower with your journemony.

Picture Time

The most fun part of this entire journey is keeping record of pictures from one month to the next. I recommend that you begin by taking a picture of your hair in its rawest state. Make sure you take a picture before and after shampooing and conditioning the hair. Include problem areas like hairline, nape, and temple areas. Be sure to take pictures with as much light as possible with a light-colored background. Print the pictures and paste them into this journal where designated, since you will be passing this down as inspiration. Otherwise, you could create a photo book of your pictures to see your progress.

Now, let's get started!

WRITE YOUR VISION FOR YOUR HAIR

_____

_____

_____

_____

_____

_____

January

Season: Cold & Dry

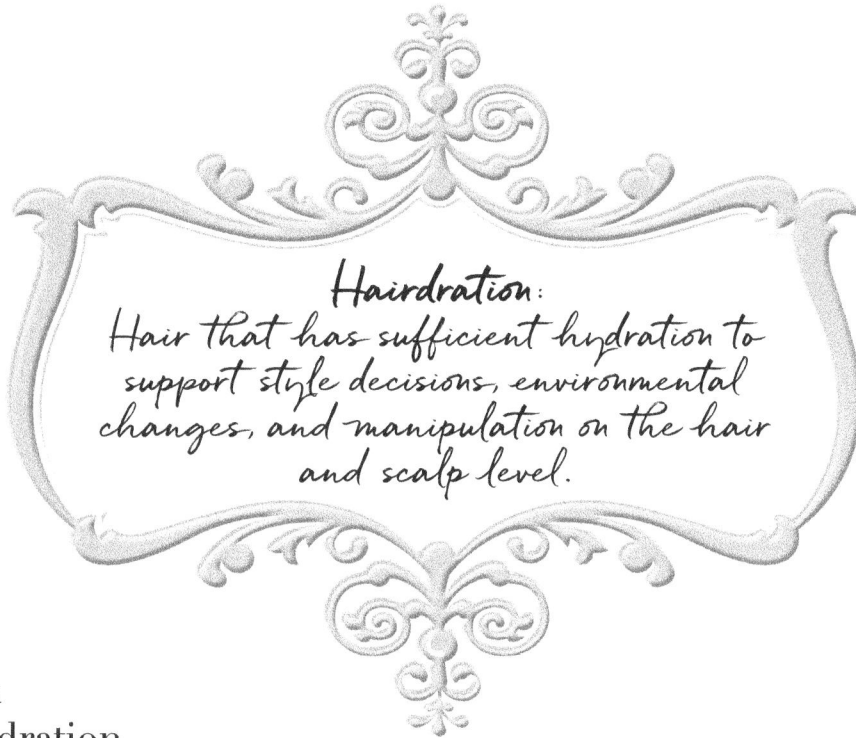

Hairdration:
Hair that has sufficient hydration to support style decisions, environmental changes, and manipulation on the hair and scalp level.

Hairdration
Week 1: Hydration
Week 2: Protective Styles
Week 3: Internal Hydration
Week 4: External Hydration
Week 5: Dehydration vs. Dryness

Seasonal Consideration:

Challenge: Keeping the hair and scalp hydrated

Decision: Style choice and hair manipulation

Goal: _____
_____
_____
_____
_____

January · Week of _____

REFLECTION

"And be renewed in the spirit of your mind" (Ephesians 4:23).

This journey will inspire a *hairadigm shift* with creative and anticipated expectations. There will be surprises and new opportunities to learn about yourself and your hair, but overall, you will be enlightened and empowered as you take the journey to discover the true potential of the MVP hair environment that's waiting to emerge. Take a moment to reflect on your vision and the plan you have created to achieve your goal. Realize that you have everything you need to make this achievable. The only hindrances you could possibly encounter will be giving up and making a decision to fall back into old *hairadigms* that led you to a place of disappointment.

RESPONSIBILITY

Mon	
Tues	
Wed	
Thu	
Fri	
Sat	
Sun	

REGIMEN: WEEK 1 HYDRATION

This is the most important topic of this month. Considering the weather and dryness created in the environment, hydration is key and will greatly benefit the hair and scalp. Just as hydration is important to your overall health, to facilitate lubrication of joints, maintain temperature, and remove waste from the body, your hair and scalp requires it for other reasons.

Daily hydration is key to supporting the strands and scalp.

I remember being told that when your hair and skin are dry, you should drink more water. Well, this is important, but not necessarily the fix-all solution. Properly hydrated hair requires more than drinking water. Drinking water supports the internal processes of the body to function, but what happens on the level of the scalp and hair is heavily dependent on the digestive system on a whole.

During winter months, hydration is needed inside and outside the body. The strands need an extra layer of protection just as your body needs layers to prevent the cold from penetrating.

Signs of Hydration

- No breakage when handling hair
- No itching of the scalp
- No frizz or static hair
- Hair is elastic and smooth to the touch

To Achieve Hydration

- You need water: half your body weight in ounces.
- Shampoo with a clarifier first to ensure the scalp and hair are clean.

- Shampoo hair weekly to prepare for deep conditioning and proper absorption of support products (proper saturation and absorption can make or break a strand).
- Condition with every shampoo—this is critical.
- Leave-in, moisture, and oil support products will buffer the strand in case there is too much manipulation between *hairgistics*.

Hairgistics

Shampoo _____

Conditioner _____

Leave-In _____

Support Product _____

Conditioning time _____

Dryer Time _____ Air dry _____

Protective Style _____

Detangle: Comb _____ Finger _____

Before

Dry	Shedding	Full		
Moist	Breaking	Frizzy		
Oily	Limp	Dull		
Stinky	Heavy	Itchy		
Tangled	Tight	Hard		

After

Dry	Shedding	Full		
Moist	Breaking	Frizzy		
Oily	Limp	Dull		
Stinky	Heavy	Itchy		
Tangled	Tight	Hard		

RELAXATION

Let me begin by saying that relaxation is necessary and not optional. Stress without relaxation equals imbalance. When the body is not balanced, disease will be welcomed into your body. The entire ecosystem was created with balance. Our bodies were created with internal checks and balances to keep everything flowing properly. Without balance, there will be disease or a signal to let you know that something is off. We must create an environment for health and wellness of the entire anatomy and physiology of the body.

A time of relaxation may include a long bubble bath with no interruptions, a time to walk in the park before 6 a.m., having a time to nap after a hard day's work, enjoying a full body massage, running a mile just for cardio, or curling up on the couch with your favorite blanket and book.

Relaxation of choice: _____

January · Week of _____

REFLECTION

"And be not conformed to this world: but be ye transformed by the renewing of your mind" (Romans 12:2)

Taking charge of any area of your life will require changes and uncomfortable adjustments. I am sure you have probably never considered that so much could be required to obtain MVP hair. It doesn't start with the strand; obtaining this environment begins in the mind. This is the part that you cannot see but has profound effects on the results of your labor. Yes, it will require a discipline that causes you to consider more than the end results. We must address the core of the issues you may have with your hair and how to find the hidden value that has yet to be discovered.

RESPONSIBILITY

Mon	
Tues	
Wed	
Thu	
Fri	
Sat	
Sun	

REGIMEN: WEEK 2 PROTECTIVE STYLES

What is a protective style? Let's begin by defining what it is not. A protective style is not a style that requires less maintenance. Protective styles require proactive style decisions. This means having or showing a strong wish to keep someone or something safe from harm. In that case, we must define what is harmful to the hair and scalp and how it needs to be protected.

Since we are endeavoring to grow MVP hair, we must also consider what healthy hair looks like. Healthy hair should be free from illness or injury. Any illness indicates that something is not performing at its expected or optimal level. Hair is protein that is designed to grow, provide coverage, and indicate your identity. MVP hair should also be elastic, meaning it should have stretch ability to avoid breakage and minimal shedding to present growth and optimal density. How the hair feels and looks causes more variables to be considered that we will address later.

For now, let's determine how to select a style that really protects how the hair maintains length and density. I realize that when most people consider a protective style, they think of braids or even a hair piece that allows for minimal manipulation and attention to the hair and scalp. Unfortunately, this is one of the worst things you can do to "protect" the hair and scalp, as it causes less attention to be given to the *hairgistics*.

Braids and hair pieces present opportunity for the hair and scalp to be neglected more than any other time because of the convenience and presentation. When considering a protective style, understand that what is most important is that the hair and scalp will still have *hairgistics* applied on a weekly or every-three-day basis if you are working out. We cannot put our hair away and think it will thrive and flourish without proper attention and care. Ultimately, every style you choose should be a protective style.

Hairgistics

Shampoo _____

Conditioner _____

Leave-In _____

Support Product _____

Conditioning time _____

Dryer Time _____ Air dry _____

Protective Style _____

Detangle: Comb _____ Finger _____

Before

Dry	Shedding	Full		
Moist	Breaking	Frizzy		
Oily	Limp	Dull		
Stinky	Heavy	Itchy		
Tangled	Tight	Hard		

After

Dry	Shedding	Full		
Moist	Breaking	Frizzy		
Oily	Limp	Dull		
Stinky	Heavy	Itchy		
Tangled	Tight	Hard		

RELAXATION

One definition for relaxation is to be free from tension and anxiety; it is recreation, enjoyment, amusement, entertainment, fun, or leisure. Only you know what causes you to feel refreshed and energized. I recommend that you choose something that is different from your normal routine in order to have the opportunity to really recreate an experience that you have not had before. I have found that doing the same relaxing activities have caused me to be so comfortable that I miss the moment and am not actually present during that activity. However, when you do something different, it will cause you to be more present and able to become fully engaged in the experience. As a result, you will also learn something new, creating new nerve and cell communication in the brain, thereby creating new memories and learning opportunities.

What relaxation experience did you choose? _____

_____

Was it new from your normal routine? _____

_____

January · Week of _____

REFLECTION

"Worrying is equivalent to being sure that you know exactly what will or will not happen based on your present observation" (Benjamin Allen Jr.).

A significant amount of our results is created by our focus and thought processes. You may find that your *hairadigm* in general needs to be adjusted. It is my endeavor to cause a *hairadigm shift* in your expectations for your hair and overall life by the end of this journal experience. Begin by determining to focus on the goal that you have set for your hair and life in general. Imagine that your focus is a seed that you are planting in a beautiful garden. Be sure to water it daily by encouraging the process and avoiding any negative thoughts (ANTs) that could come to eat the plants. Remember that patience is key, and rest in the fact that your body is created to involuntarily grow hair from the inside out. Your responsibility is to make sure that your inside thoughts are conducive for MVP hair. You are built to grow, and growth is a constant part of your makeup. Be encouraged—you have a long way to grow!

RESPONSIBILITY

Mon	
Tues	
Wed	
Thu	
Fri	
Sat	
Sun	

REGIMEN: WEEK 3 INTERNAL HYDRATION

Yes, just as hair growth and vitality originates from the inside out, hydration does as well. Most have been told about the importance of drinking water to improve hydration; however, there is much more to consider when trying to properly hydrate the internal workings of the body to facilitate MVP hair.

While considering this subject, I began to observe my clients and the condition of their hair based on their water consumption. What I found was very interesting. I did not observe a difference in the condition of the hair based on how much water was consumed. This led me to begin researching how nutrition affects hair growth and vitality. Even from birth, a child's head of hair grows without weekly salon appointments and deep conditioning. It even grows without the consumption of pure water. Therefore, there is a set program that is created inside of every human being to produce and grow hair.

So how do some maintain "optimum density and length" while others seem to struggle? As we grow and develop, the body requires more nutrition based on the demands that are placed on the body. This varies from one individual to the next and has to be determined based on the requirements of activity and stamina. All body systems are supported by protein production. Without going too deep, we need protein, and protein requires essential fatty acids for the skin. An essential amino acid cannot be made by the body, hence having to come from food and supplements.

To ensure that your internal hydration is sufficient, a balanced meal plan that includes protein, essential fatty acids, and water are a good place to start. We will discuss nutrition is greater detail later.

Hairgistics

Shampoo _____

Conditioner _____

Leave-In _____

Support Product _____

Conditioning time _____

Dryer Time _____ Air dry _____

Protective Style _____

Detangle: Comb _____ Finger _____

Before

Dry	Shedding	Full		
Moist	Breaking	Frizzy		
Oily	Limp	Dull		
Stinky	Heavy	Itchy		
Tangled	Tight	Hard		

After

Dry	Shedding	Full		
Moist	Breaking	Frizzy		
Oily	Limp	Dull		
Stinky	Heavy	Itchy		
Tangled	Tight	Hard		

RELAXATION

Another definition of relaxation is recreation or rest, especially after a period of work. Sometimes, you can find it hard to relax because of internal issues that have not been addressed. You may want to consider finding a quiet place where you either record yourself releasing any cares or responsibilities onto a voice recorder, or if you prefer to write, purchase a new journal to empty out all that has been floating around in your head that will not allow you to rest. Afterward, decide to treat yourself to a "lazy day" where you decide to only do what you absolutely want to do and only if you decide to do anything. Schedule your lazy day and record it in the responsibility section of this journal.

January · Week of _____

REFLECTION

If your mind is needed to do everything else that is to be accomplished, shouldn't it be the part of your body that gets the most care and consideration so it can continue to perform as needed?

Your mind has many responsibilities, and normally, more responsibilities means more compensation. How will you choose to compensate yourself for being responsible for your hair and health?

_____

_____

You deserve to be appreciated and recognized for the worth and inspiration that you bring to your surroundings. Although we as humans may not be able to please everybody, I guarantee you that there is someone else that values your existence and contribution to life. You must take time to reflect on as many experiences as possible that either yielded physical compensation or appreciation for you just being you. Take time to reflect on what you have been appreciated for by others, and those things that have yet to be acknowledged should be recognized and celebrated by you. It's all right to encourage yourself too!

RESPONSIBILITY

Mon	
Tues	
Wed	
Thu	
Fri	
Sat	
Sun	

REGIMEN: WEEK 4 EXTERNAL HYDRATION

External hydration specifically and strategically addresses the strand and scalp. There is a part of the anatomy of the scalp called the *acid mantel* that functions to keep the scalp balanced and free from bacteria if the proper environment is created. If the scalp is properly cleaned with shampoos that do not disturb the acidity of the skin, the acid mantel will release a substance called sebum to maintain the proper moisture of the scalp.

Now I understand that we were taught to oil the scalp so it would not be dry, but this was misguided information. The scalp has been created to be self-sufficient, and as long as we maintain a clean and uncompromised environment, the scalp should not itch. By the same token, oil, just like water, cannot hydrate the scalp, or anything else for that matter. Oil is used to seal whatever state the scalp or strand is already in. Therefore, if the scalp is dry, the oil will only make the scalp feel more lubricated as it seals in the current state of dryness. The lubrication gives a false sense of change in the way the scalp feels but does not change the actual condition of the scalp. Same with the strand: oil seals the current state, while moisture, which normally contains some water content, will hydrate the strand, increasing elasticity and guarding against breakage.

Hairgistics

Shampoo _____

Conditioner _____

Leave-In _____

Support Product _____

Conditioning time _____

Dryer Time _____ Air dry _____

Protective Style _____

Detangle: Comb _____ Finger _____

Before

Dry	Shedding	Full		
Moist	Breaking	Frizzy		
Oily	Limp	Dull		
Stinky	Heavy	Itchy		
Tangled	Tight	Hard		

After

Dry	Shedding	Full		
Moist	Breaking	Frizzy		
Oily	Limp	Dull		
Stinky	Heavy	Itchy		
Tangled	Tight	Hard		

RELAXATION

Relaxation is also defined as the loss of tension in a part of the body, especially in a muscle when it ceases to contract.

When it comes to true relaxation, I love having massages, preferably by my husband. But if he is not available, a foot massage is my other preference. I realize that everybody is not comfortable with having someone rub on them, but if you are, please schedule a massage, even if it's just a foot massage or a pedicure where reflexology is offered. I guarantee, it could change your life if you get the right masseuse.

January · Week of _____

REFLECTION

"To whom much is given much is required" (Luke 12:48).

When I first heard this verse, I did not understand its significance in my life. Sometimes you may feel like you are not given much of anything or may not even ask for much. Well, whether you realize it or not, there is more being provided for us than we may have the focus to appreciate. This became a reality for me during a mission trip to the Bahamas. I could really see just how much was given based on my socioeconomic environment. There are things that we take for granted, like immediate access to water that can be used for brushing your teeth. Take time to Google less fortunate environments and see just how much has been given that is not always available to others. It is at this point that you may find a greater appreciation for the responsibilities that come with much that is given.

RESPONSIBILITY

Mon	
Tues	
Wed	
Thu	
Fri	
Sat	
Sun	

REGIMEN: WEEK 5 DEHYDRATION VS. DRYNESS

Dehydration is the state of losing water whereas dryness concerns the outward manifestation of something that lacks or needs moisture. I just learned and you probably have not considered that drinking water does not change your skin from being dry to moist. Yes, that's correct; no matter how much water you drink, it will not change the condition of your skin. As mentioned in the previous week, the skin needs vital nutrition to continue proper function of the body.

Research shows that ideal body water is 50–60 percent for men and 45–60 percent for women. Therefore, drinking water may support the water content that you already have or help to replenish water loss from the body, but it will not change the condition of your skin or hair without additional support products and maintenance techniques that support the viability of your hair and scalp. We will speak more about water contribution to the body in the nutrition section of the journal. For now, focus on incorporating proper nutrition and support products to ensure that the scalp and strands are properly supported to avoid dryness, itching, and breakage.

Hairgistics

Shampoo _____

Conditioner _____

Leave-In _____

Support Product _____

Conditioning time _____

Dryer Time _____ Air dry _____

Protective Style _____

Detangle: Comb _____ Finger _____

Before

Dry	Shedding	Full		
Moist	Breaking	Frizzy		
Oily	Limp	Dull		
Stinky	Heavy	Itchy		
Tangled	Tight	Hard		

After

Dry	Shedding	Full		
Moist	Breaking	Frizzy		
Oily	Limp	Dull		
Stinky	Heavy	Itchy		
Tangled	Tight	Hard		

RELAXATION

The action of making a rule or restriction less strict is another definition of relaxation. Sometimes we place demands on ourselves that create unnecessary stress to our already hectic lifestyles. For example, I remember a time when I desired to reach out to so many people a day, just to encourage them or check on them. Well, although it was a desire in my heart to do it and it was a good idea, I applied pressure on myself to do so many per day. Ultimately, no one was expecting it, and I hadn't even made any promises to anyone to fulfill this idea. Therefore, I decided to release myself from doing five per day and reduced my commitment to one per day when I began to feel overwhelmed.

Revisit your release journal and see if there are any responsibilities that you could either restructure, delegate, or release from your schedule of self-inflicted expectations for as long as you desire—to relax from it. Replace that time with whatever you desire to do in that moment.

Journal what you released and what replaced that time that will contribute to your time of relaxation.

_____

_____

_____

_____

_____

Journemony Time

Express your thoughts about the journey so far and what inspired you to
take the challenge.

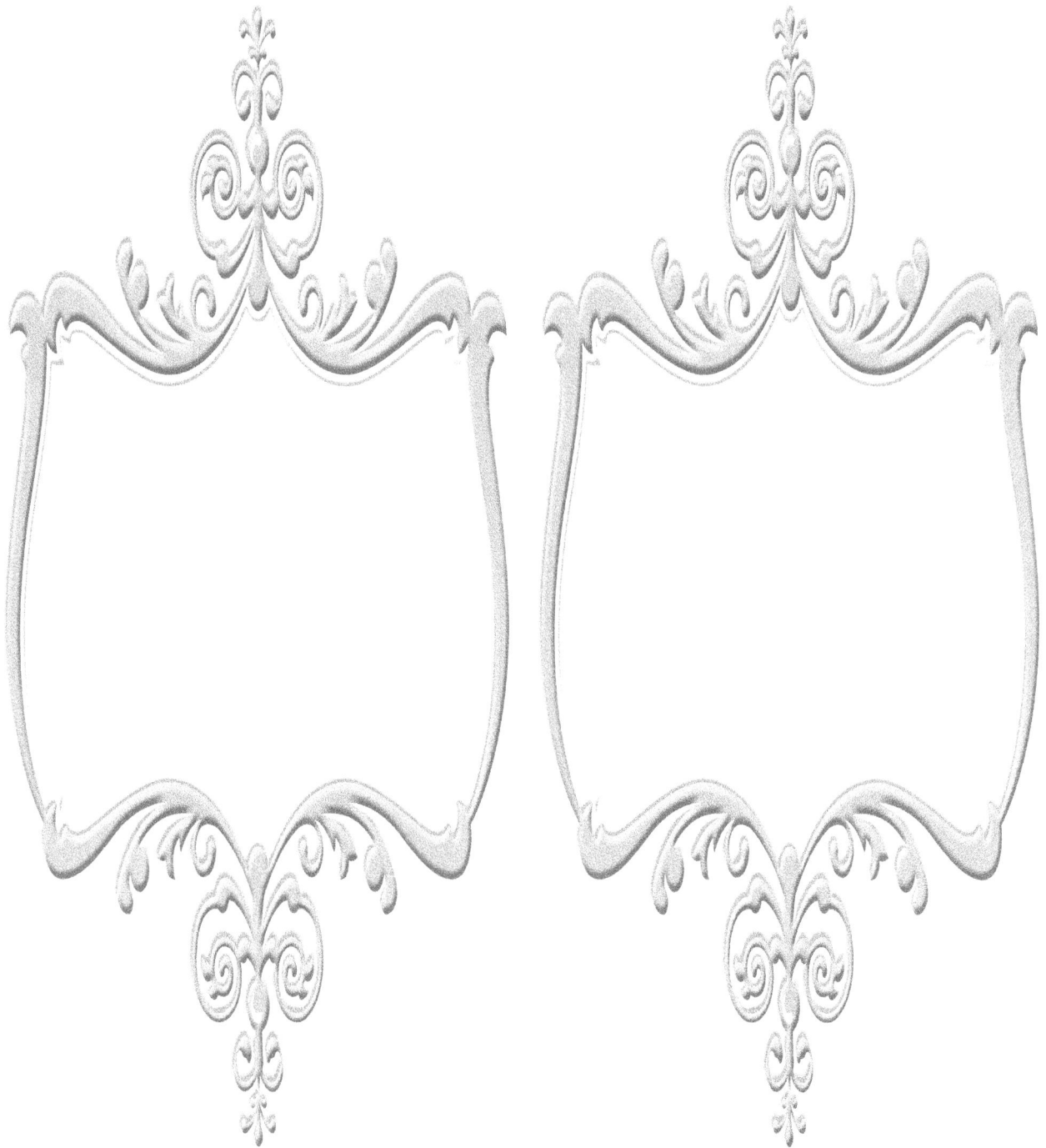

Picture Time

February _____

Season: Cold & Dry

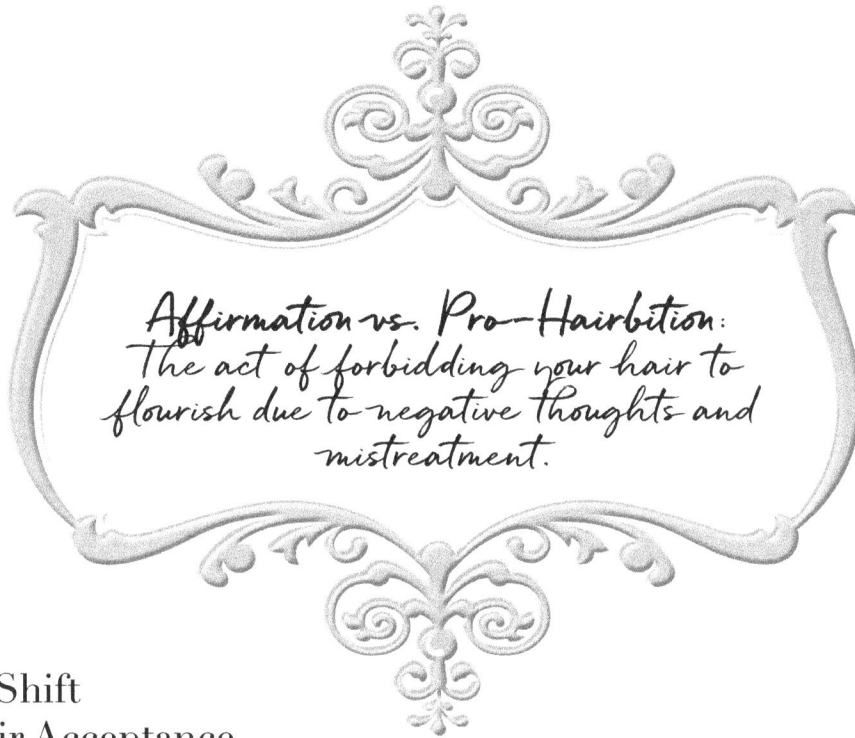

Affirmation vs. Pro-Hairbition:
the act of forbidding your hair to
flourish due to negative thoughts and
mistreatment.

Hairadigm Shift
Week 1: Hair Acceptance
Week 2: Hair Affirmation
Week 3: Hair Support & Cover
Week 4: Hair Relation-tips

Seasonal Consideration:

Challenge: Keeping the hair and scalp hydrated

Decision: Style choice and hair manipulation

Goal: _____
_____
_____
_____
_____

February · Week of _____

REFLECTION

Identity: Who are you? Does your hair really define who you are as a person?

_____

_____

I believe you should reconsider allowing something as fragile as hair to become an identifier of your qualities and worth. Yes, it provides a way to observe similarities amongst race and ethnicity at times, but does it really say much else about how you contribute to the lives of others?

RESPONSIBILITY

Mon	
Tues	
Wed	
Thu	
Fri	
Sat	
Sun	

REGIMEN: WEEK 1 HAIR ACCEPTANCE

An unfortunate amount of focus has been given to hair and how it defines us. This should be refocused into having an appreciation for the opportunity to reveal creativity and responsibility for a part of God's creation. I have met so many people in this industry that constantly have disdain for their hair. Sometimes it takes years for a person to grow to love their own hair in its natural state. It is amazing how influenced we can be by others' acceptance before our own. Should it really take someone else to approve of our hair before we deem it worthy to be appreciated? Determine in your heart and mind that your hair is acceptable, and appreciate its natural or chemically modified state. Then, watch how much easier it will respond to your care. Consider the brains beneath the hair before allowing the hair to control the brain.

Hairgistics

Shampoo _____

Conditioner _____

Leave-In _____

Support Product _____

Conditioning time _____

Dryer Time _____ Air dry _____

Protective Style _____

Detangle: Comb _____ Finger _____

Before

Dry	Shedding	Full		
Moist	Breaking	Frizzy		
Oily	Limp	Dull		
Stinky	Heavy	Itchy		
Tangled	Tight	Hard		

After

Dry	Shedding	Full		
Moist	Breaking	Frizzy		
Oily	Limp	Dull		
Stinky	Heavy	Itchy		
Tangled	Tight	Hard		

RELAXATION

If you are not accustomed to handling your own hair and are trying it for the first time, you may find that it is a little stressful to think about the responsibility that you have taken on in addition to all of the other things that your life requires. If this is you, think of an ideal setting that you could create on your own to make the environment more suitable for relaxation while treating your hair. You may want to consider transforming your bathroom into a spa area. Dim the lights while in the shower, light your favorite candle, and play soft music during this week.

February · Week of _____

REFLECTION

"So shall my word be that goeth forth out of my mouth: it shall not return unto me void, but it shall accomplish that which I please and it shall prosper in the thing whereto I sent it" (Isaiah 55:11).

Word power: Did you know that sound is vibrations, and vibrations cause movement? Well, without giving a full quantum physics lesson, understand that sound is created to cause a response. When you give a command to someone, you expect a response, and when that response is not experienced, it is determined that something is wrong or out of alignment or agreement. Have you noticed if your hair is responding to what you have been speaking about it?

_____

_____

Begin to take notice of your *hairadigm* and reconsider your word choices and expectations.

RESPONSIBILITY

Mon	
Tues	
Wed	
Thu	
Fri	
Sat	
Sun	

REGIMEN: WEEK 2 HAIR AFFIRMATION

In light of the scripture reflection, we must consider what we have been speaking about our hair. Have you been speaking words of affirmation or *pro-hairbition*? Most people only speak what they see and experience concerning their hair, and as a result, they will attract the same unwanted experiences. Affirmation can only begin with a change of thought. We must begin to think differently about our hair before we can speak differently and obtain new results. Begin to speak the opposite of any negative thoughts or do not speak anything at all. Next, find something that you are pleased with about your hair and begin speaking that in place of nothing at all. Instead of, "My hair is so thick and unmanageable," you could convert that to, "I have optimal density that requires thorough nourishment and careful manipulation." Thinking positive yields to speaking positive, and speaking positive yields to believing positive.

Hairgistics

Shampoo _____

Conditioner _____

Leave-In _____

Support Product _____

Conditioning time _____

Dryer Time _____ Air dry _____

Protective Style _____

Detangle: Comb _____ Finger _____

Before

Dry	Shedding	Full		
Moist	Breaking	Frizzy		
Oily	Limp	Dull		
Stinky	Heavy	Itchy		
Tangled	Tight	Hard		

After

Dry	Shedding	Full		
Moist	Breaking	Frizzy		
Oily	Limp	Dull		
Stinky	Heavy	Itchy		
Tangled	Tight	Hard		

RELAXATION

You would be surprised how relaxing it could be to complete a task that you have been meaning to finish for some time. When you leave a task unfinished, it lingers in your mind, causing a sense of disturbance. This removes the balance that accommodates a relaxed state of being. You may decide that the task is too much for you and needs to be delegated, or you may just need to solicit help. Either way, the experience of completing the task will not only provide a sense of accomplishment but also a sense of relief.

February · Week of _____

REFLECTION

"But if a woman have long hair, it is a glory to her: for her hair is given her for a covering" (1 Corinthians 11:15).

For those who have resolved that long hair is not your preference, it is your right to prefer whatever you desire for your hair. Pay close attention to the word *if* in this passage. *If* implies a conditional clause, which means that what comes after the *if* is conditional. Therefore, for those that desire or have long hair, you will have more sufficient covering or protection from outside exposure. Hair has more purpose than to just make you feel better about the way you look and present yourself to others. It was actually created to provide protection or covering of the scalp.

RESPONSIBILITY

Mon	
Tues	
Wed	
Thu	
Fri	
Sat	
Sun	

REGIMEN: WEEK 3 HAIR COVER & SUPPORT

Depending on the environment, you should determine the type of covering needed to protect the hair. In the winter, the hair should always be supported by products that provide moisture and promote elasticity. This is where your leave-in conditioners and moisturizers play a great role in hairgistics. When exposing the hair to cold, wind, and rain, appropriate covering should be applied. Keep in mind that just as you dress your hair for bed, a proper covering should also be applied during the day. Do not allow your hair or hairline and nape to come in contact with any material that will absorb your moisture. Either find hats and scarves that have silk or satin texture on the inside or use an individual scarf or turban, depending on your style, to protect the hair from materials like cotton and wool. This is very important to consider when wrapping the neck with scarves as well, because over time, the nape will experience unnecessary breakage due to the drying effect and contact the scarf has with the nape.

Hairgistics

Shampoo _____

Conditioner _____

Leave-In _____

Support Product _____

Conditioning time _____

Dryer Time _____ Air dry _____

Protective Style _____

Detangle: Comb _____ Finger _____

Before

Dry	Shedding	Full		
Moist	Breaking	Frizzy		
Oily	Limp	Dull		
Stinky	Heavy	Itchy		
Tangled	Tight	Hard		

After

Dry	Shedding	Full		
Moist	Breaking	Frizzy		
Oily	Limp	Dull		
Stinky	Heavy	Itchy		
Tangled	Tight	Hard		

RELAXATION

Relaxation is in the mind of the beholder. Did you know that the mind is just as powerful as reality? Studies have shown that the mind does not really know what is real and what isn't. This is why some people can read or meditate on a particular symptom and experience it. Think about the times you have been around someone that was sick, and although you were just fine, you began to think about the possibility of catching whatever they had. More often than not, most people allow their brains to receive that vision and begin to experience similar symptoms. On the other hand, we cannot feel very well and come into contact with someone with more energy and vitality and pick up the same vibes, finding ourselves better after contact.

So where is your mind this week? Could we possibly try to focus on being on a remote island, away from every care that we have no control to change anyway, and enjoy thinking beyond our reality?

February · Week of _____

REFLECTION

To thine own hair be true.

Your hair in its natural state is a part of your individuality, not how you style or color or manipulate it into something else. Think about how exciting it would be if each month you looked forward to seeing the expression of how the hair emerges out of the scalp. What if it didn't mean that it is almost time for a relaxer or that the smoothness of the hair would begin to fade? What if we truly begin to embrace the relationship that our hair originally desires to develop with us? Based on how it expresses itself from the scalp, it is speaking and telling us just what it needs. What if we listened to our hair and stopped listening to what everyone else is saying that our hair needs? Wouldn't this be more rewarding to know that not only are you appreciating your hair just as it grows, but you also have the ability to respond to its needs and cultivate a relationship to achieve MVP hair?

RESPONSIBILITY

Mon	
Tues	
Wed	
Thu	
Fri	
Sat	
Sun	

REGIMEN: WEEK 4 HAIR RELATION-TIPS

How to relate to your hair.

Determine what works for you: natural, relaxed, braided, short, long. What is your preference?

Determine what works for your hair based on your ability to respond to what it needs. You may have time constraints or a lack of interest in taking care of your hair. Consider the season and schedule of your life before making decisions about how you will wear your hair. Did you know that a synonym for *wear* is "service" or "value," and the capacity for withstanding continuous use without damage? This tip is key because our first desire should be "to do no harm and protect at all cost."

Just as you desire for others to treat you a certain way in relationships, there are boundaries that your hair expresses when harm has been experienced. If the heat is too hot, the hair will melt. If the comb is too strong, the hair will break. There are many ways that the hair is speaking, and everyone's hair requires different things based on its individuality. Fine hair has to be handled more carefully than course hair, but both have to be handled with care. Become more aware of what your hair is telling you, and determine how to relate to it by prioritizing what will cause it to flourish over what you may desire to only please yourself or others.

Hairgistics

Shampoo _____

Conditioner _____

Leave-In _____

Support Product _____

Conditioning time _____

Dryer Time _____ Air dry _____

Protective Style _____

Detangle: Comb _____ Finger _____

Before

Dry	Shedding	Full		
Moist	Breaking	Frizzy		
Oily	Limp	Dull		
Stinky	Heavy	Itchy		
Tangled	Tight	Hard		

After

Dry	Shedding	Full		
Moist	Breaking	Frizzy		
Oily	Limp	Dull		
Stinky	Heavy	Itchy		
Tangled	Tight	Hard		

RELAXATION

If you have been following the journal and participating as prescribed, you should have created a new pathway or circuitry in your brain to relax at least one day of the week. If you continue to desire to relax, your body will demand that you relax. It will remind you with adverse symptoms if something is in opposition to your relaxed state of being. This will only serve as an indication that something is not in alignment with your original desire. Remember the mind is intelligent enough to know when something is out of order because it has recorded your thoughts and actions and is trained to follow a program that has already been set. When this program is detoured, the body will not follow without a fight. Be advised that your own body is the best accountability partner you may have ever had.

From this point on, it is your responsibility to schedule and create opportunities for relaxation for the sake of your overall health and well-being. I will remind you of its importance, but you must use your creativity based on your needs to create environments for relaxation. It is my desire that you eventually incorporate a time of relaxation daily and just before bed.

Journemony Time

Dear Loved One,

If I could give one word of advice concerning how to love yourself, it
would be . . .

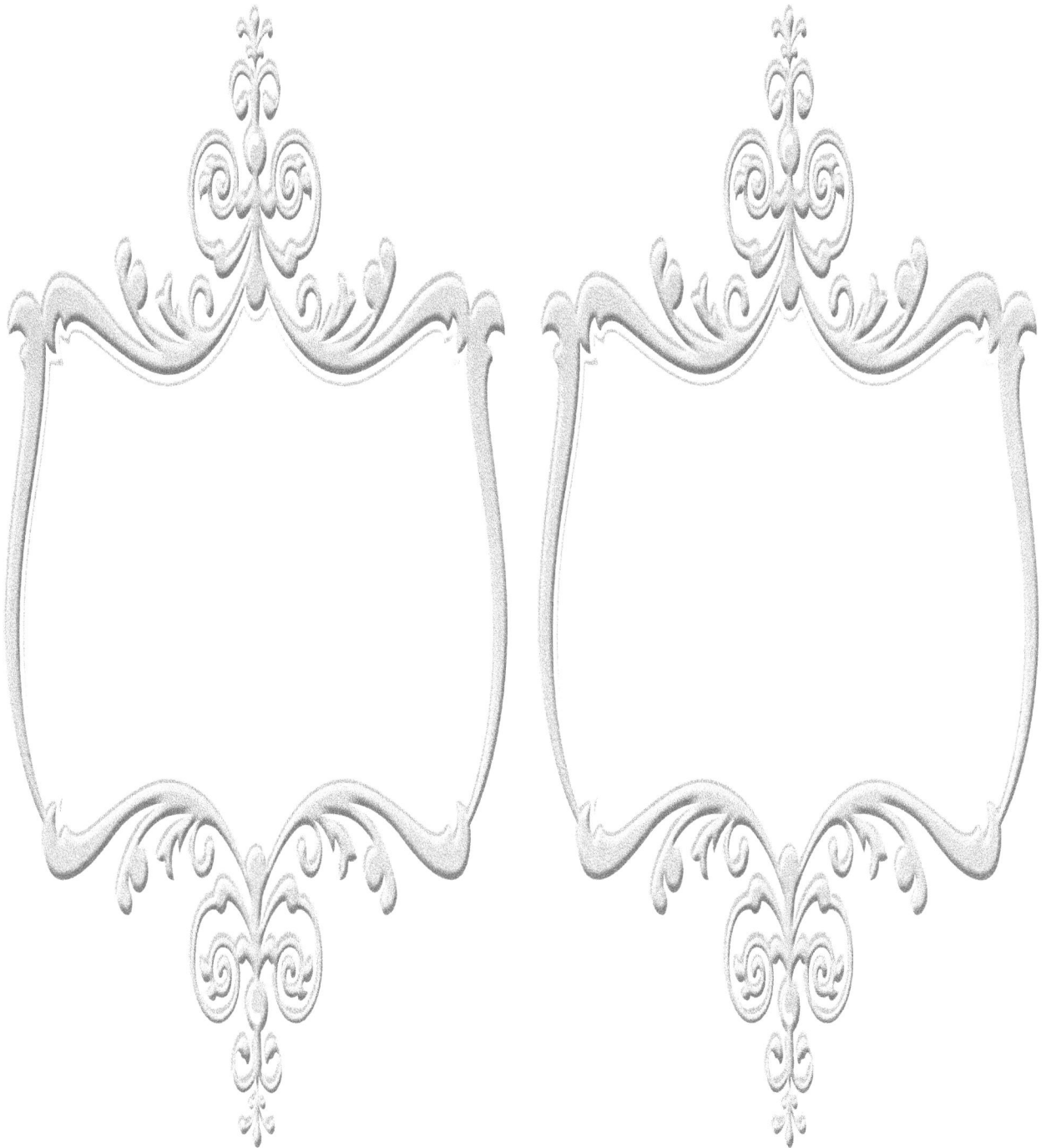

Picture Time

March _____

Season: Cool & Windy

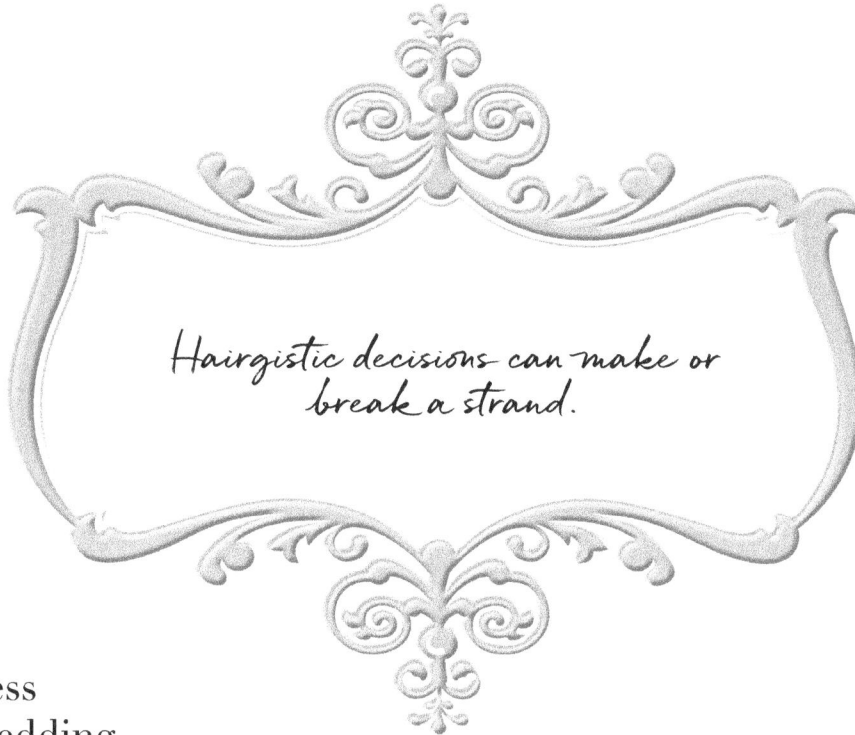

Hairgistic decisions can make or break a strand.

Hair Madness
Week 1: Shedding
Week 2: Detangling
Week 3: Manageability
Week 4: Style Decisions

Seasonal Consideration:

Challenge: Keeping the hair and scalp moisturized and tangle free. Become aware of what is shed hair vs. breakage.

Decision: Style choice and hair manipulation

Goal: _____

_____

_____

_____

_____

March · Week of _____

REFLECTION

"But even the very hairs of your head are numbered. Fear not therefore; ye are of more value than many sparrows" (Luke 12:7).

The sparrow was a bird offered in the Old Testament by the very poor, signifying that if God takes the time to acknowledge their existence, being less valuable in quality than other sacrifices, your hair being unnecessary to sustain life is just as important to God as any other part of the body and regarded as equally valuable and worthy of protection. If He has taken the time to number the strands, He is acknowledging His attention to each strand as well. Whatever He creates has value and purpose and should be equally appreciated by us as well.

RESPONSIBILITY

Mon	
Tues	
Wed	
Thu	
Fri	
Sat	
Sun	

REGIMEN: WEEK 1 SHEDDING

Shedding is a casting off of something from a normal process. It is natural and normal for hairs to shed 50–100 strands per day. Anything over this parameter is considered abnormal and referred to as *telogen effluvium*. *Telogen* refers to the stage of natural shedding the hair experiences during its hair growth cycle. *Effluvium*, a word used in the 1600s, means "a flowing out of air," relating to the way the hair would be more likely to release from the scalp. This process of shedding does not include hair that has been forced by manipulation.

A good way to determine if your hair has released naturally or is broken is by examining the ends of the strand. If you can see a little ball on the tip of the strand, this indicates shedding. If you cannot see a little ball on either end, this indicates breakage. Experiencing more than 50–100 strands does not mean you have excessive shedding. You could be experiencing breakage.

Hairgistics

Shampoo _____

Conditioner _____

Leave-In _____

Support Product _____

Conditioning time _____

Dryer Time _____ Air dry _____

Protective Style _____

Detangle: Comb _____ Finger _____

Before

Dry	Shedding	Full		
Moist	Breaking	Frizzy		
Oily	Limp	Dull		
Stinky	Heavy	Itchy		
Tangled	Tight	Hard		

After

Dry	Shedding	Full		
Moist	Breaking	Frizzy		
Oily	Limp	Dull		
Stinky	Heavy	Itchy		
Tangled	Tight	Hard		

RELAXATION

Have you ever noticed while riding in the car or sitting at the computer that you are naturally holding a position of tension? Well, I realized that my back would be slightly curved as if I was anticipating having to move abruptly or catch myself quickly. My husband noticed that he would curl his toes while at the computer. I believe that it takes extra focus to notice when you think you are relaxing but not fully relaxing due to voluntary tension positions. To really know how each part of your body should feel when it is fully relaxed, begin by applying deliberate tension to each body part. For example, tighten your fist for about ten seconds as tight as you can. Then release it. This is your normal conscious state of relaxation. Try it on your legs, back, stomach, buttocks, neck, face, and any other area that you can apply tension or stress to, and release the tension to feel what state you should maintain unconsciously.

March · Week of _____

REFLECTION

"And be not entangled again with the yoke of bondage" (Galatians 5:1).

Up to this point you have reconsidered your *hairadigm*. Unfortunately, just having an idea is not powerful enough to become reality. We also must have experience to support the idea before it can become a part of our belief system. However, sometimes we do not allow enough time to experience what is needed to permanently change how we view certain things. Here is where I want you to be determined to hold on to the *hairadigm shifts* and allow time for your hair to transform based on your new thoughts and *hairgistics*. What has taken years to develop will still require time to experience a difference. Thankfully, it only takes one year to experience 6 inches of new growth, so this turnaround will produce desired results much sooner than what it took for you to receive undesirable results. Do not allow yourself to look back and retreat to what has been comfortable or familiar because one year is taking too long to experience a new you.

RESPONSIBILITY

Mon	
Tues	
Wed	
Thu	
Fri	
Sat	
Sun	

REGIMEN: WEEK 2 DETANGLING

The possibility of unnecessary hair loss results more from improper detangling than any other part of the styling system. Any movement between strands creates the potential for tangling, especially if the root of the strand is different from the shaft and ends. This is my favorite part of styling because it allows me to use my organizational skills on a head of hair, which creates an environment for more control. Detangling is really a proactive process that requires focus and organization. It begins as soon as you are preparing to dress your hair for bed and continues throughout the week until the next shampoo. To detangle the hair requires you to avoid opportunities for tangles in the first place. For example, the hair should never be put in a position where the roots and strands are allowed to congregate without being organized.

Detangling should occur daily, before shampooing and after conditioning, if needed. A comb should only be used after a manual finger detangle has been applied in order to ensure that any shed hair is completely released from the strands. It is also important to gently comb or finger comb the hair away from the scalp perpendicular to the head instead of down with the natural flow of gravity. Gravity will encourage the heaviness of the natural strength of your hand to possibly break through a tangle that was missed during the manual detangling process. By combing the hair out instead of down through the remaining density, you will be less likely to break the hair that has direct contact with the comb.

In addition to repositioning your hand to comb out instead of down, imagine that the comb is being used as a tool to give your hair a Swedish massage. How careful you desire for someone to caress you should be kept in mind while massaging your hair with the comb. Be sure to always section the hair to avoid becoming overwhelmed, and try creating a relaxing environment during the detangling session to relax the whole body as much as possible.

Never detangle when you are in a hurry; it could be detrimental and lead to breakage. If you notice that a lot of hair is coming out, apply the strand observation discussed in the previous week to determine if you are breaking your hair off or releasing shed hair during your detangling process. Adjust your *hairgistics* based on your observation.

Hairgistics

Shampoo _____

Conditioner _____

Leave-In _____

Support Product _____

Conditioning time _____

Dryer Time _____ Air dry _____

Protective Style _____

Detangle: Comb _____ Finger _____

Before

Dry	Shedding	Full		
Moist	Breaking	Frizzy		
Oily	Limp	Dull		
Stinky	Heavy	Itchy		
Tangled	Tight	Hard		

After

Dry	Shedding	Full		
Moist	Breaking	Frizzy		
Oily	Limp	Dull		
Stinky	Heavy	Itchy		
Tangled	Tight	Hard		

RELAXATION

When you are experiencing stress, the body responds by releasing chemicals that indicate if you are in a fight or flight situation, something that we should only experience when in imminent danger, like being chased by a wild animal or under the pressure of a mass murderer holding you hostage in your home. This causes the muscles to become tense, heart and respiration rates increase, and other parts of the body feel fatigue.

More importantly, the body is also wired to focus on more of a survival mode of operation than immune response. So, when we are stressed, the body thinks that our life is in danger and takes away from the body's ability to heal, thereby resulting in a compromised or less alert immune system. This is how we can experience sickness during times of chronic stress; the body is so busy trying to stay alive that it doesn't provide the focus to maintain normal health conditions. Think about it: if a wild animal is about to eat you, the sore throat is irrelevant until the danger has passed. So please take your time of relaxation, even if you just appreciate the fact that you do not live in the rain forest with exotic wild animals.

March · Week of _____

REFLECTION

"The thoughts of the diligent tend only to plenteousness; but of every one that is hasty only to want" (Proverbs 21:5).

Diligent means having or showing care and conscientiousness in your work or duties. Pay attention to your hair this week with more focus than before. See what you may not have noticed that was overlooked. Is your hair responding to the product that you are using, or does it seem to be drying faster than you need it to? How about your detangling technique; are you losing less hair since you have more instruction and experience with this process?

_____

_____

Listen to your hair and watch it increase and respond positively to your efforts as you take your time and observe its unique characteristics.

RESPONSIBILITY

Mon	
Tues	
Wed	
Thu	
Fri	
Sat	
Sun	

REGIMEN: WEEK 3 MANAGEABILITY

When something is manageable, it is capable of being controlled. This begins with a decision of style preference and time management. How much time do you have to properly take care of your hair, and what style is convenient for you to produce within your time constraints? All hair is manageable with proper instruction and technique, which is determined by how you decide to wear your hair. Generally, most hair styles other than dreads or locks need some type of conditioning and support product to maintain a smooth, vibrant expression. Hair also requires proper dressing for bed—satin or silk bonnets that do not apply tension or friction to the edge of the hairline.

Hairgistics

Shampoo _____

Conditioner _____

Leave-In _____

Support Product _____

Conditioning time _____

Dryer Time _____ Air dry _____

Protective Style _____

Detangle: Comb _____ Finger _____

Before

Dry	Shedding	Full		
Moist	Breaking	Frizzy		
Oily	Limp	Dull		
Stinky	Heavy	Itchy		
Tangled	Tight	Hard		

After

Dry	Shedding	Full		
Moist	Breaking	Frizzy		
Oily	Limp	Dull		
Stinky	Heavy	Itchy		
Tangled	Tight	Hard		

RELAXATION

Are you the type of person that can't relax because you are an overachiever or not able to treat yourself because nothing is ever good enough? Well, when you tense up consistently, this can lead to muscle aches, headaches, backaches, and eventually fatigue. The symptoms that result due to a lack of relaxation could contribute to you being less productive, experiencing more frustration and even less relaxation. Refuse to continue the cycle, and start recognizing when you need to relax.

March · Week of _____

REFLECTION

"Multitudes, multitudes in the valley of decision" (Joel 3:14).

A *decision* is a conclusion reached after consideration. As you reflect on your life and *hairloom*, be sure to take time each week to make decisions that will benefit not only you but the next generation. Often we imagine that what we do will only truly affect us; but after further consideration, we will realize that every decision we make has an effect on someone else, whether we know it or not. Your smile while in the grocery line could provide hope for someone who began to believe that there was no one else in the world who cares enough to make eye contact and acknowledge their existence. Be more aware of how vital you are as a human being, and it will have a greater effect on how you see others and decide to interact with your present environment.

RESPONSIBILITY

Mon	
Tues	
Wed	
Thu	
Fri	
Sat	
Sun	

REGIMEN: WEEK 4 STYLE DECISIONS

Hair styles come in three categories: up, down, or a combination of both. Styles that are down require daily detangling, whether natural or chemically treated. While up styles require support products and attention to the shape of the style as well as the flow of the style.

Style decisions should never be based on what someone else suggests for how you should look. Style decisions should be based on how well you can maintain that style without having to compromise your MVP status. For example, a smooth roller set should not be chosen when it's time for a relaxer. A tighter set or twist style should be chosen to avoid trying to match the new growth with the straighter style expression. Up styles are preferable over down when it's time for a relaxer. This allows for the hair to rest and not have to experience unnecessary handling that could lead to breakage at the line of demarcation, where the new growth and chemically relaxed hair meet.

Hairgistics

Shampoo _____

Conditioner _____

Leave-In _____

Support Product _____

Conditioning time _____

Dryer Time _____ Air dry _____

Protective Style _____

Detangle: Comb _____ Finger _____

Before

Dry	Shedding	Full		
Moist	Breaking	Frizzy		
Oily	Limp	Dull		
Stinky	Heavy	Itchy		
Tangled	Tight	Hard		

After

Dry	Shedding	Full		
Moist	Breaking	Frizzy		
Oily	Limp	Dull		
Stinky	Heavy	Itchy		
Tangled	Tight	Hard		

RELAXATION

In addition to the expected symptoms of a lack of relaxation, you could also experience the following:

- Pain and disease
- Indecisiveness
- Energy depravation
- More opportunities for mistakes
- Mental, physical, and emotional exhaustion
- Focus deficiency
- Less satisfaction
- Isolation and depression

Therefore, before you go to the doctor to have some of these symptoms misdiagnosed, try taking some time off and relaxing.

Journemony Time

Dear Loved One,

As the years fly by and I see all of the changes of perspective that I have experienced concerning my hair, I want to encourage you to . . .

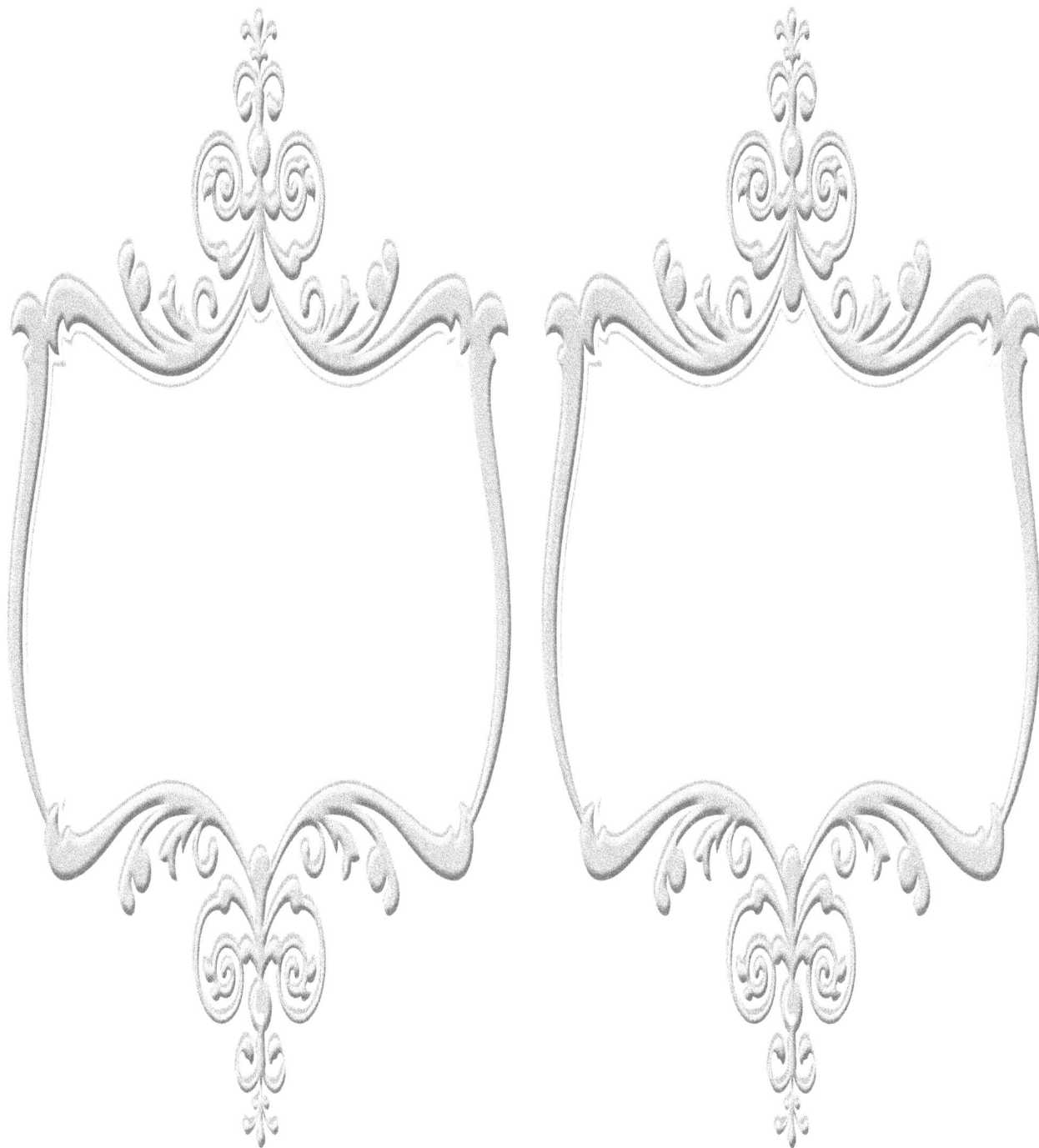

Picture Time

April _____

Season: Rain & Humidity

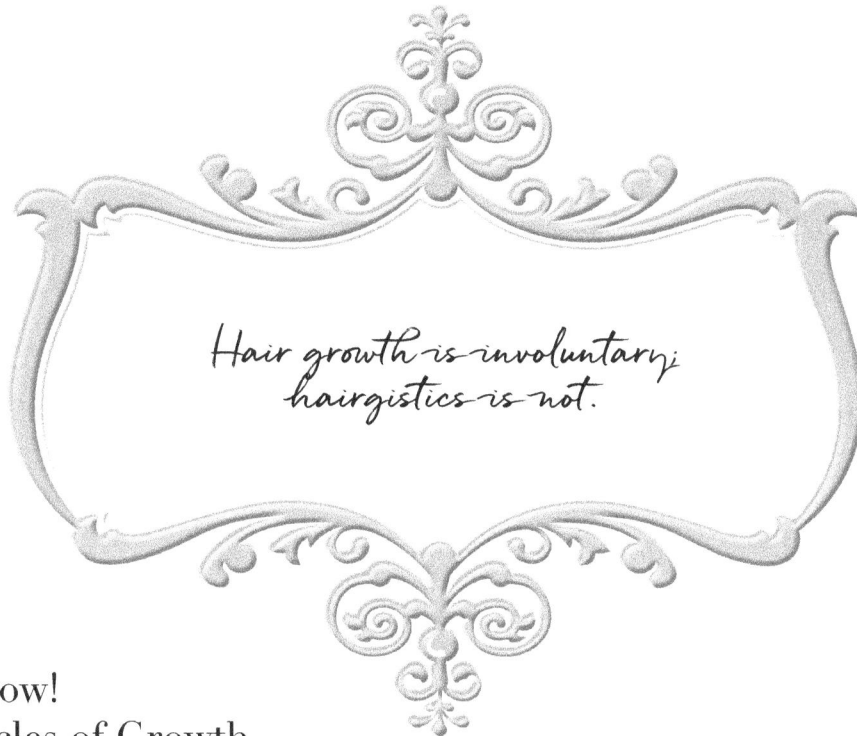

Hair growth is involuntary; hairgistics is not.

Hair We Grow!
Week 1: Cycles of Growth
Week 2: Anagen, Catagen, Telogen
Week 3: Strand Layers
Week 4: Product Decisions

Seasonal Consideration:

Challenge: Keeping the hair from frizzing

Decision: Style choice and hair manipulation

Goal: _____
_____
_____
_____
_____

April · Week of _____

REFLECTION

"And he shall be like a tree planted by the rivers of water that bring forth fruit in season" (Psalm 1:3).

This scripture reminds me of how hair grows. When the proper environment is set, MVP hair will emerge. What type of environment are you allowing in your life that may not be conducive for growth and prosperity in your life? Take time to journal the areas that are beneficial and not so beneficial. Take each item and decide what would need to happen for change to occur.

_____

_____

_____

_____

_____

RESPONSIBILITY

Mon	
Tues	
Wed	
Thu	
Fri	
Sat	
Sun	

REGIMEN: WEEK 1 CYCLES OF GROWTH

There are three main cycles of hair growth. The design of God manifests in many ways through cycles. A cycle represents a circle that has no beginning and no end. Such is the way hair seems to emerge from the scalp. The strand you see comes from beneath the *epidermis* (scalp) from the *dermis* (layer beneath the epidermis). It all begins with the heart of your hair, known as the *derma papilla*, hence why it is important to love your hair and be nice to it! This is the area that connects blood flow from every other part of your body to the strand.

Through a very interesting series of connections and stimulations, the hair follicle is attaching, taking root, and creating cells that continue to build one on top of the other until it emerges as a chemically bonded group of amino acids called protein (normally known as keratin) through the epidermis. It is very similar to that of the way a seed is planted, takes root, is watered and nourished, and forms into the stem to push through the soil and emerge above ground. The beauty of the strand, unlike the plant, is that it cannot be completely uprooted without surgical means, so it always has a connection with the heart to continue to receive and produce what it needs to emerge as a strand.

This happens while three distinct phases are taking place: anagen, catagen, and telogen (ACT) phases. Thankfully, each strand is on its own cycle, because if it wasn't, we could possibly grow and lose all of our hair at the same time—and that would be devastating.

Hairgistics

Shampoo _____

Conditioner _____

Leave-In _____

Support Product _____

Conditioning time _____

Dryer Time _____ Air dry _____

Protective Style _____

Detangle: Comb _____ Finger _____

Before

Dry	Shedding	Full		
Moist	Breaking	Frizzy		
Oily	Limp	Dull		
Stinky	Heavy	Itchy		
Tangled	Tight	Hard		

After

Dry	Shedding	Full		
Moist	Breaking	Frizzy		
Oily	Limp	Dull		
Stinky	Heavy	Itchy		
Tangled	Tight	Hard		

RELAXATION

How has the knowledge of how important relaxation is to the whole health of the body affected your perspective of taking time for yourself?

_____

_____

_____

April · Week of _____

REFLECTION

"To everything there is a season and a time to every purpose under heaven, a time to be born and a time to die" (Ecclesiastes 3:1-2).

In the fabric of creation, we see cycles and patterns through nature, and the hair is no different. There are also times in your life where, at one point, a situation felt very important, and later it seemed unimportant. This is all a part of life and our ability to adapt, grow, and prosper. There has to be a growing stage and a pruning stage. What areas of your life may be overdue for pruning because it no longer has the ability to benefit your growth and development?

_____

_____

RESPONSIBILITY

Mon	
Tues	
Wed	
Thu	
Fri	
Sat	
Sun	

REGIMEN: WEEK 2 ANAGEN, CATAGEN, TELOGEN

The anagen phase is the most favorable phase for most to learn about because it indicates the possibility of growth for at least 2–7 years straight. However, this is also a very critical time because whatever you are growing will also stay with you for the same amount of time if it doesn't break or get cut off.

On average, if you can successfully maintain all of the length without cutting or breaking the hair, you should be able to grow 6 inches per year, and 2–7 years is approximately 30 inches of hair (otherwise known as *waist length*, for most). Think about how long you have been on the earth and have had hair that was not being cut on a regular basis. If you have never maintained a haircut and have allowed your hair to grow, you should at least have 24–30 inches by now, and if you don't, it's because you have constantly created an environment for the hair to experience weak areas along the shaft which is prone to breakage.

The catagen phase is very hard to measure and lasts about 1–3 weeks because, like all of the other phases, each strand is in its own stage at any particular time, which means not all strands will grow or shed at the same time. Catagen gives the strand an opportunity to rest from all of its hard work as it prepares to release—what is better known as the telogen or shedding phase.

The telogen phase allows the strand to disconnect from the inner workings of the cycle and release in the form of a shed hair. Remember, a shed hair will have a little ball on the end indicative of the remaining cells that were sitting inside of the follicle at the time of the telogen phase. This is when growth stops to prepare to leave the dermis. The telogen phase is promising because it reminds me of forgiveness or the chance to release and start over.

If you decided to wear braids for an extended amount of time without *hairgistics*, the hair will become very dry and porous, giving the appearance of a zigzag pattern along the strand because of the dehydration of the shaft. Over time, those same strands that were compromised during that time will eventually shed and begin to present new growth, which means a new strand and a new opportunity to express or present something different.

Hairgistics

Shampoo _____

Conditioner _____

Leave-In _____

Support Product _____

Conditioning time _____

Dryer Time _____ Air dry _____

Protective Style _____

Detangle: Comb _____ Finger _____

Before

Dry	Shedding	Full		
Moist	Breaking	Frizzy		
Oily	Limp	Dull		
Stinky	Heavy	Itchy		
Tangled	Tight	Hard		

After

Dry	Shedding	Full		
Moist	Breaking	Frizzy		
Oily	Limp	Dull		
Stinky	Heavy	Itchy		
Tangled	Tight	Hard		

RELAXATION
What are some things you have learned about how you prefer to relax?

_____

_____

April · Week of _____

REFLECTION

"The spirit of a man will sustain his infirmity" (Proverbs 18:14).

Did you know that you are not just what you physically see and touch, or even just a ball of feelings and emotions? You are also a solid combination of chemicals, hormones, and organic matter. How you choose to express who you want others to see is totally within your God-given free will and power. What you think affects your perception and what you perceive affects your belief system. Make sure you have more than just the surface information to draw conclusions about yourself and others. It could mean the difference between the life and death of a relationship.

RESPONSIBILITY

Mon	
Tues	
Wed	
Thu	
Fri	
Sat	
Sun	

REGIMEN: WEEK 3 STRAND LAYERS

Although a strand is very fragile, it too has more depth than what meets the eye. Three layers—the cuticle, cortex, and medulla—all come together to create the strand you know to be a hair. Each layer has a different responsibility and can prove vital to the longevity of a strand.

The *cuticle* is like the skin of a piece of fruit: it determines what is allowed in and out. Let's call it the "gate keeper." While the *cortex* is the processing center for what is allowed in and out. It either receives the chemical and converts it to something desirable or it reflects something that you may not have expected, depending on how cooperative your previous condition is with the new process. Lastly, the *medulla* is a hollow tube that you may or may not find, depending on the texture and type of strand. What is important for you to know is that the cortex is the part that provides the most strength to the entire strand—about 80 percent. If this layer is in its optimal state and is uncompromised, you will be more likely to keep your hair and obtain length. I will discuss this more in October (Week 3 Strand Integrity).

Hairgistics

Shampoo _____

Conditioner _____

Leave-In _____

Support Product _____

Conditioning time _____

Dryer Time _____ Air dry _____

Protective Style _____

Detangle: Comb _____ Finger _____

Before

Dry	Shedding	Full		
Moist	Breaking	Frizzy		
Oily	Limp	Dull		
Stinky	Heavy	Itchy		
Tangled	Tight	Hard		

After

Dry	Shedding	Full		
Moist	Breaking	Frizzy		
Oily	Limp	Dull		
Stinky	Heavy	Itchy		
Tangled	Tight	Hard		

RELAXATION

If you could go back in time, what event would you erase from your life that caused a ripple effect of a lack of relaxation?

_____

_____

_____

_____

April · Week of _____

REFLECTION

"Commit thy works to the Lord and thy thoughts shall be established" (Proverbs 16:3).

In any opportunity to make decisions, there must always be a foundation upon which to build. Once you have set your goals and vision for your hair or life in general, your decisions should be made to accommodate the vision. The responsibility required to support your vision and goals should not be neglected because of your everyday routine or unexpected opportunities that present themselves after you have established where you are headed. Since you have determined to commit to taking care of your hair unlike ever before, you should allow no one to deter you based on their vision or foundation that they set for themselves. That would cause instability, and without a firm foundation, your vision cannot be established or stand firm.

RESPONSIBILITY

Mon	
Tues	
Wed	
Thu	
Fri	
Sat	
Sun	

REGIMEN: WEEK 4 PRODUCT DECISIONS

I must admit that the verdict is still out on what constitutes the market's perfect product line. Unfortunately, this is a trial and error opportunity to explore. I will say that you want your products to be skin friendly, and some even recommend that you only use on your hair and scalp what you would put *in* your body. This suggestion is taking hair care to another level, and after a while, I do believe that is where we are headed, considering all of the ingredients that are being eliminated from products due to toxicity. Overall, we are still a very intelligent design and have endured way more than the drying effects of a high pH-formulated shampoo or conditioner. Therefore, decide what works best for not only how your hair feels and looks but also the condition of your scalp and how it feels and looks. Furthermore, if you don't remember anything else, keep in mind that no hair care product can cure damaged hair; it can only treat and make the hair look, feel, or behave differently until you decide to cut the damaged area.

Hairgistics

Shampoo _____

Conditioner _____

Leave-In _____

Support Product _____

Conditioning time _____

Dryer Time _____ Air dry _____

Protective Style _____

Detangle: Comb _____ Finger _____

Before

Dry	Shedding	Full		
Moist	Breaking	Frizzy		
Oily	Limp	Dull		
Stinky	Heavy	Itchy		
Tangled	Tight	Hard		

After

Dry	Shedding	Full		
Moist	Breaking	Frizzy		
Oily	Limp	Dull		
Stinky	Heavy	Itchy		
Tangled	Tight	Hard		

RELAXATION

What would you tell your loved one about relaxation, and what would you be willing to contribute to their journey of learning to relax daily?

_____

_____

_____

_____

Journemony Time

Dear Loved One,

There are several stages of growth and development that we experience during this journey called life. Equally important is our growth and development in relationships. Always be sure to consider . . .

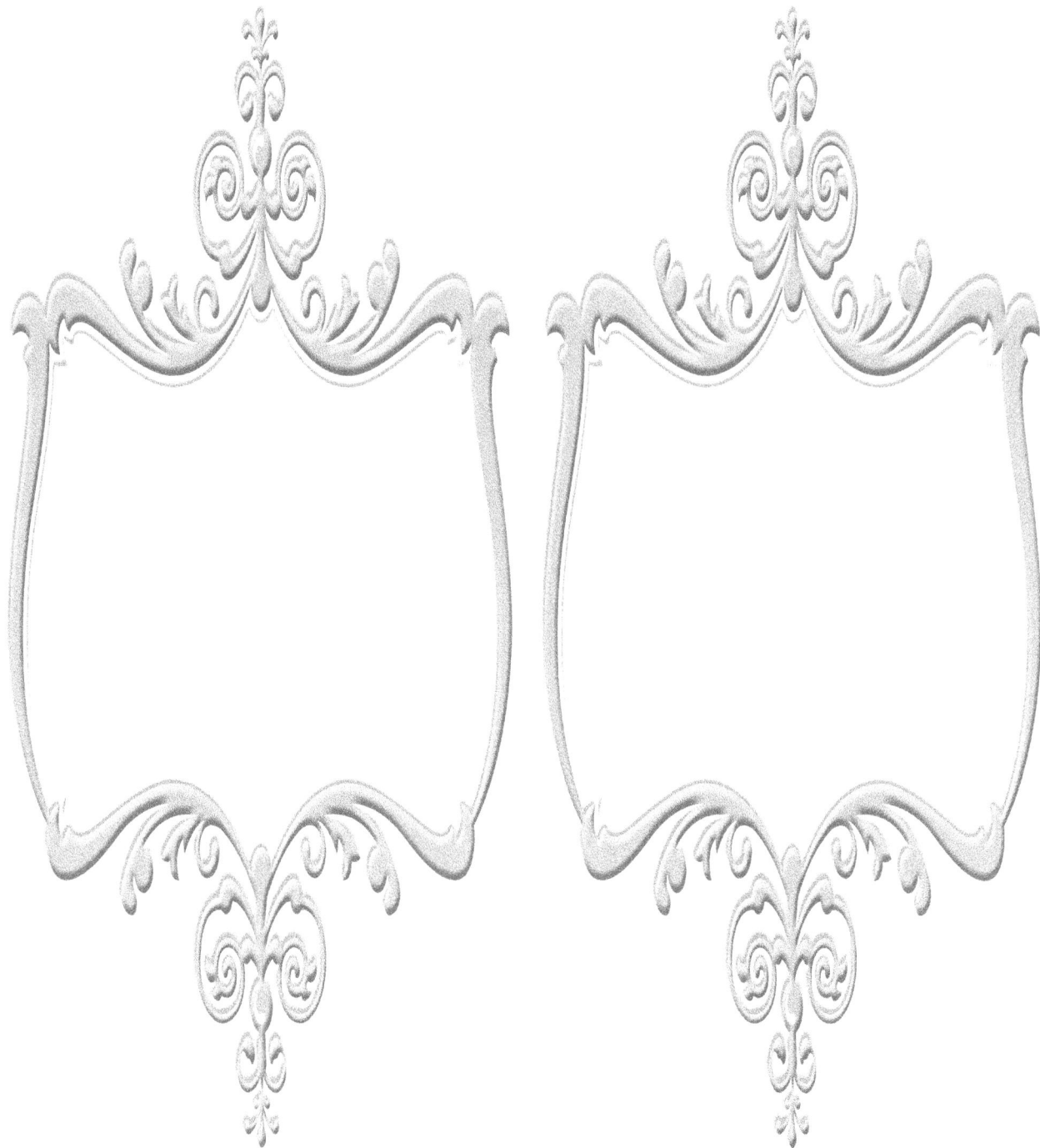

Picture Time

May

Season: Warm Days, Cool Nights

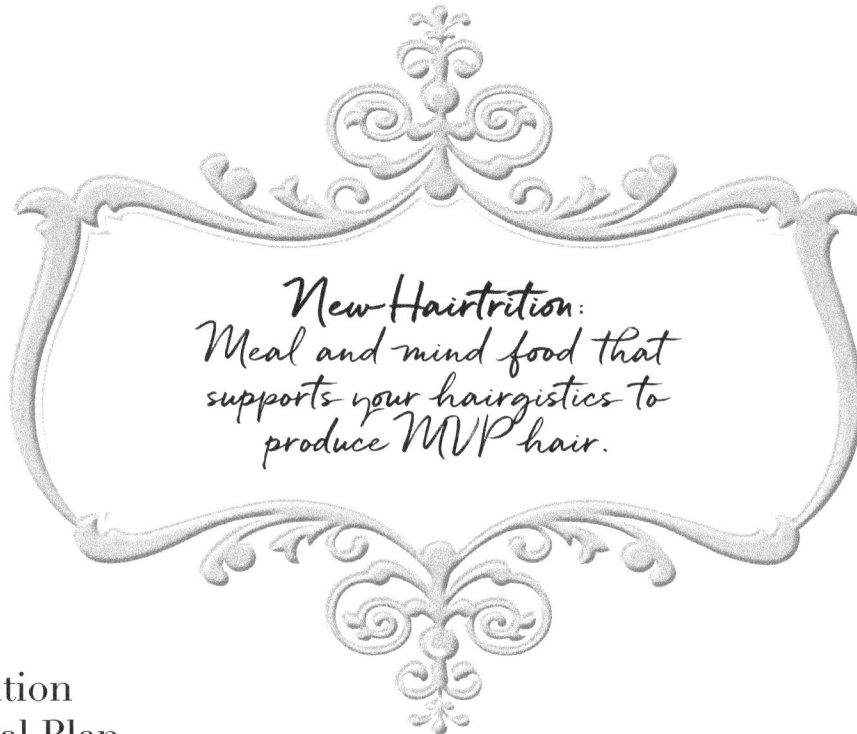

New Hairtrition:
Meal and mind food that
supports your hairgistics to
produce MVP hair.

New Hairtrition
Week 1: Meal Plan
Week 2: Supplements
Week 3: Water
Week 4: Hair Food Suggestions

Seasonal Consideration:

Challenge: Keeping the hair covered from the different elements

Decision: Style choice and hair manipulation

Goal: _____

_____

_____

_____

_____

May · Week of _____

REFLECTION

"Man shall not live by bread alone" (Matthew 4:4).

We must understand that the natural part of you is given in order to understand the spiritual part of you. What does your appetite consist of? Are you satisfied with the same things all of the time, or do you prefer variety?

_____

_____

Either way, we must take the time to consider why we prefer what we prefer and determine if it is beneficial for our natural and spiritual growth and development. We all need sustenance, and it needs to be more than just the bread you are accustomed to eating.

RESPONSIBILITY

Mon	
Tues	
Wed	
Thu	
Fri	
Sat	
Sun	

REGIMEN: WEEK 1 MEAL PLAN

Regardless of what type of meal plan you choose, I have yet to find a healthy plan that will benefit the entire body that doesn't consist of a variety of categories and choices. For example, the food chart from elementary school suggested the different serving amounts for sufficient daily intake. Well, although the chart has been revised based on the body's needs regarding health, exercise programs, and age, you still have to have protein, fats, and carbohydrates—and meat, vegetables, and starch is the normal combination to consider.

Since this is a hair journal, I will leave the nutritional research up to you to determine what your individual body needs. Just keep this in mind: you are made of proteins, chemicals, hormones, and liquid. Therefore, what you are made of is greatly affected by what you consume and what you think about what you consume. Food choices are personal, and their effects are very subjective in the whole scheme of things.

Listen to your body, and based on your goals for your health, determine how what you consume makes you feel first, not how it tastes. Then begin the investigation of what works for you. Next, find out what the food has to offer that will benefit the health of your body. Don't just eat for taste or cravings. Did you know that when you crave sweets, it means you are deficient in protein? And when you crave fatty, greasy foods, you need healthy fats like Omega-3, -6, -9? These substitutes will shut cravings completely off by filling the gaps.

Hairgistics

Shampoo _____

Conditioner _____

Leave-In _____

Support Product _____

Conditioning time _____

Dryer Time _____ Air dry _____

Protective Style _____

Detangle: Comb _____ Finger _____

Before

Dry	Shedding	Full		
Moist	Breaking	Frizzy		
Oily	Limp	Dull		
Stinky	Heavy	Itchy		
Tangled	Tight	Hard		

After

Dry	Shedding	Full		
Moist	Breaking	Frizzy		
Oily	Limp	Dull		
Stinky	Heavy	Itchy		
Tangled	Tight	Hard		

RELAXATION

Avoid considerations of food for your relaxation opportunity. You should consume food to live—not live to consume. Certain foods only produce and send certain chemical messages that affect the chemistry of the body. Therefore, you are not really relaxing while eating because digestion is working during this process. You are actually just tricking your body to feel a certain way while consuming that food. Since food consumption can lead to other issues, let's only use it for what it is intended, and that is to give the body the fuel it needs to be healthy and have energy.

May · Week of _____

REFLECTION

"And beside this, giving all diligence, add to your faith virtue, and to virtue knowledge and to knowledge temperance and to temperance patience and to patience godliness and to godliness brotherly kindness and to kindness charity" (2 Peter 1:5-7).

I commend you for taking the challenge to create a *hairloom*; and I am sure you are learning a lot about yourself that you probably had not considered before now. Whether you experience a lesson or a blessing, life is a learning process that has opportunities for trial and error, and it will continue to carry you as long as you keep learning and refuse to give up. My spiritual mentor says that there are no mistakes unless you mis-take the lesson that is attached to the experience. Become a lifelong learner and you will continue to grow and develop into who you are created to be.

RESPONSIBILITY

Mon	
Tues	
Wed	
Thu	
Fri	
Sat	
Sun	

REGIMEN: WEEK 2 SUPPLEMENTS

After all of the strategic meal planning, we still have opportunity to make sure we have all of the things that the body needs to produce the energy and biological processes necessary to sustain life. These are called *supplements*, and they are very tricky because the only way you can fully benefit from a supplement is to already have the substance that you are trying to supplement in your meal plan—hence the term *supplement*. A supplement is something that completes or enhances something else when added to it. Sorry, it doesn't replace or fill an empty place, it only adds. Be careful with self-diagnosing because you could overdose and cause unnecessary changes in your body when taking too many supplements. If not completely sure, a prenatal vitamin is normally safe enough for regular supplementation.

Hairgistics

Shampoo _____

Conditioner _____

Leave-In _____

Support Product _____

Conditioning time _____

Dryer Time _____ Air dry _____

Protective Style _____

Detangle: Comb _____ Finger _____

Before

Dry	Shedding	Full		
Moist	Breaking	Frizzy		
Oily	Limp	Dull		
Stinky	Heavy	Itchy		
Tangled	Tight	Hard		

After

Dry	Shedding	Full		
Moist	Breaking	Frizzy		
Oily	Limp	Dull		
Stinky	Heavy	Itchy		
Tangled	Tight	Hard		

RELAXATION

Speaking of supplements, don't you think it's time to consider adding a little more time to your relaxation period? If you have scheduled 1 day a week, go on and let your hair down this week and take a couple of extra hours just to supplement your relaxation time.

May · Week of _____

REFLECTION

Just as the body needs water for life chemistry to flow properly, purpose and guidance is needed in order for your life to flow as it has been designed. Reconnect with the Creator and seek guidance for how to flow.

RESPONSIBILITY

Mon	
Tues	
Wed	
Thu	
Fri	
Sat	
Sun	

REGIMEN: WEEK 3 WATER

We are made of at least 70 percent water, and water helps things to flow properly. No one wants to get stuck, be stuck, or have anything stuck inside of the body that needs to move out. So think about this when you have issues drinking water: it's like turning on a garbage disposal full of food with no running water. Although it may break the food down, it will have a harder time than with the assistance of the water to further dissolve the particles. Furthermore, eventually something may even get stuck inside and start to stink. So just be mindful of washing down your insides with the recommended "half your body weight in water" (in ounces) measurement. I have read that a glass of water first thing in the morning even helps the blood to begin circulating and causes phlegm from congestion to loosen.

Note: If you are 160 lbs., drink 80 oz. per day. That's it! Watch how much better you feel and flow.

Hairgistics

Shampoo _____

Conditioner _____

Leave-In _____

Support Product _____

Conditioning time _____

Dryer Time _____ Air dry _____

Protective Style _____

Detangle: Comb _____ Finger _____

Before

Dry	Shedding	Full		
Moist	Breaking	Frizzy		
Oily	Limp	Dull		
Stinky	Heavy	Itchy		
Tangled	Tight	Hard		

After

Dry	Shedding	Full		
Moist	Breaking	Frizzy		
Oily	Limp	Dull		
Stinky	Heavy	Itchy		
Tangled	Tight	Hard		

RELAXATION

Relaxation is also a way to keep things flowing and balanced. Have you noticed that after you relax, you can think more clearly and have more energy?

May · Week of _____

REFLECTION

"As new born babes desire the sincere milk of the word that ye may grow thereby" (1 Peter 2:2).

In order to obtain different results, change is necessary. Some of our choices, whether food, disciplines, or relationships, need to be adjusted so that we can create an environment conducive for health and healing. Just as babies require a clean environment and pure, natural sustenance, we too should consider revisiting the basics or former choices that foster a simpler approach to life.

RESPONSIBILITY

Mon	
Tues	
Wed	
Thu	
Fri	
Sat	
Sun	

REGIMEN: WEEK 4 HAIR FOOD SUGGESTIONS

Protein, carbohydrates, fats, vitamins, supplements, water, fruits, vegetables, nuts and seeds.

There is no cure-all combination that will guarantee the perfect environment for "healthy hair and scalp care" for every individual across the globe. Therefore, it is up to you to make the best choices for your health care needs, because all of us require different nutritional sustenance based on our activities, lifestyle, weight, age, and other genetic factors.

Maintain a food journal when you decide to find what works best for the overall care of your entire body. It may require adjustments along the way, but at least you will learn what truly benefits you nutritionally instead of just eating for pleasure and causing more harm than health.

Hairgistics

Shampoo _____

Conditioner _____

Leave-In _____

Support Product _____

Conditioning time _____

Dryer Time _____ Air dry _____

Protective Style _____

Detangle: Comb _____ Finger _____

Before

Dry	Shedding	Full		
Moist	Breaking	Frizzy		
Oily	Limp	Dull		
Stinky	Heavy	Itchy		
Tangled	Tight	Hard		

After

Dry	Shedding	Full		
Moist	Breaking	Frizzy		
Oily	Limp	Dull		
Stinky	Heavy	Itchy		
Tangled	Tight	Hard		

RELAXATION

As I was writing this journal, it seemed like the relaxation portion began to come faster and faster as I addressed each month. I pray that you are truly investing in this part of the journal and enjoying taking care of yourself with a more holistic approach.

Journemony Time

Dear Loved One,

Although medical records consider family history when making assessments of health care needs, remember that you can be proactive and create an environment for health and healing by . . .

Picture Time

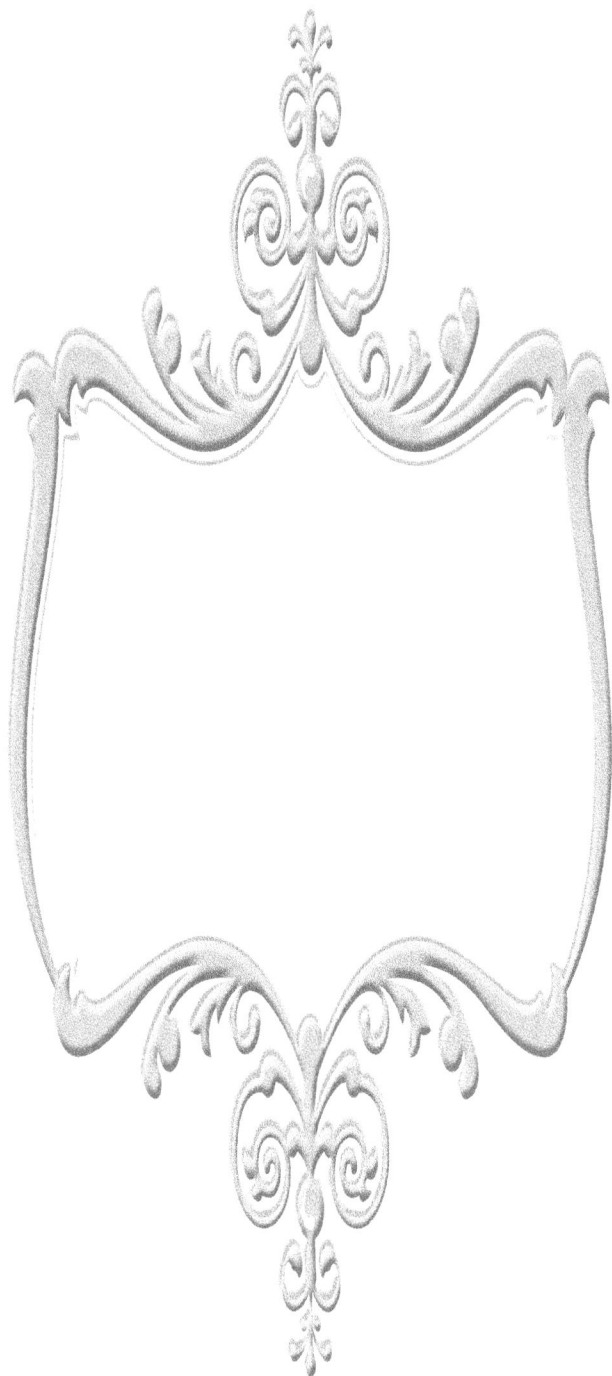
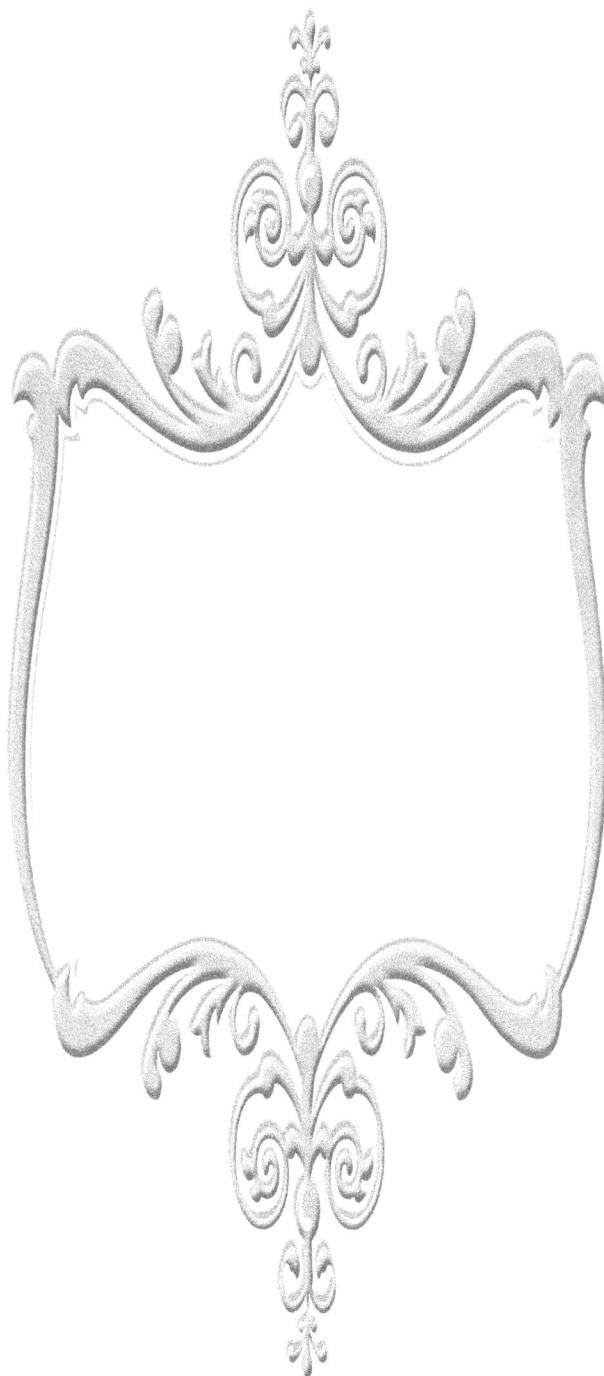

June

Season: Hot

MVP Hair:
Manageable, Viable, Protected

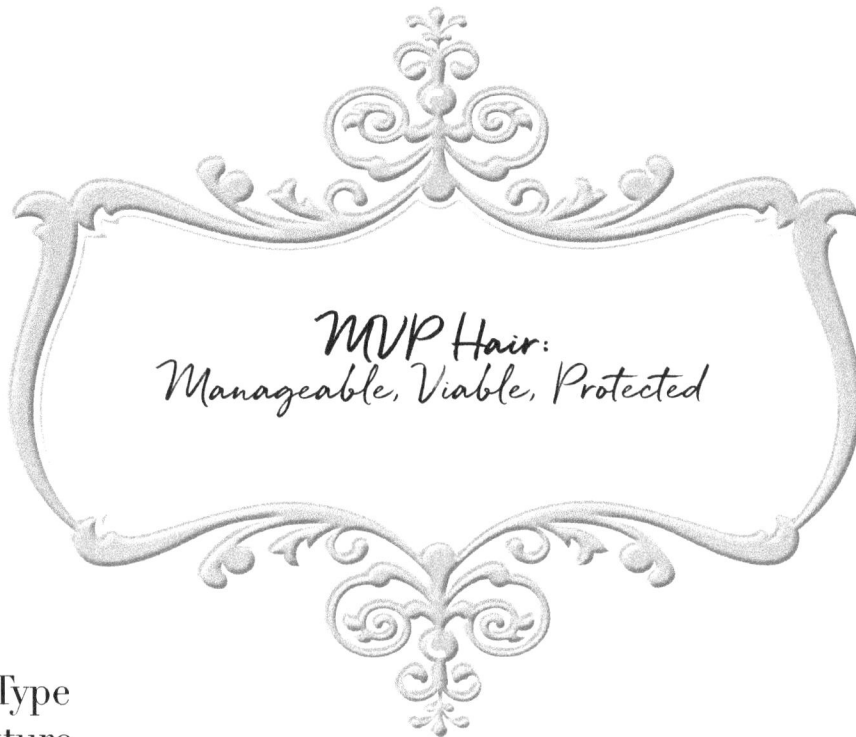

Texture vs. Type
Week 1: Texture
Week 2: Type
Week 3: Transitioning
Week 4: Porosity

Seasonal Consideration:

Challenge: Keeping the hair and scalp cool

Decision: Style choice and hair manipulation

Goal: _____

_____

_____

_____

_____

Hairloom

June · Week of _____

REFLECTION

"Whatsoever things are true, honest, just, pure, lovely, are of good report . . . think on these things" (Philippians 4:8).

What is your *hairadigm*? Have you ever had a time that you were totally satisfied?

_____

_____

If not, you may be experiencing a case of *pro-hairbition* syndrome, the act of forbidding your hair to flourish due to negative thoughts and mistreatment. There has to be something that you can appreciate about your hair even if it's just the fact that you have some on your head. Always look a little deeper and be thankful for even the smallest things in life, because it, like a seed, could turn into something greater than you could ever imagine.

RESPONSIBILITY

Mon	
Tues	
Wed	
Thu	
Fri	
Sat	
Sun	

REGIMEN: WEEK 1 TEXTURE

The terms *good hair* or *bad hair* should never be used to describe how your hair expresses its individuality. Instead of subjecting it to your category of the level of difficulty in how it responds to *hairgistics*, you should consider keeping it simple. Just look at the shape of the strand. Is it straight, wavy, curly, or spiral? I commend the more specific classifications that allow further detail, but unfortunately, most heads do not have the same texture throughout the entire head. Therefore, it's safe to say that knowing the texture may not help you to determine how to care for the hair because how you care for your hair depends on the condition of the strand, not the shape of the strand.

Heat is heat, chemical is chemical, products are products. How much you use should be based on instructions and on what your hair needs, which can only be determined by performing the service. Just because something worked on the "YouTuber" doesn't mean it's going to work on you because your hair looks similar.

Hairgistics

Shampoo _____

Conditioner _____

Leave-In _____

Support Product _____

Conditioning time _____

Dryer Time _____ Air dry _____

Protective Style _____

Detangle: Comb _____ Finger _____

Before

Dry	Shedding	Full		
Moist	Breaking	Frizzy		
Oily	Limp	Dull		
Stinky	Heavy	Itchy		
Tangled	Tight	Hard		

After

Dry	Shedding	Full		
Moist	Breaking	Frizzy		
Oily	Limp	Dull		
Stinky	Heavy	Itchy		
Tangled	Tight	Hard		

RELAXATION

Stay on course and remember to allow your hair an opportunity to relax also. If you always have it tied up around the house, because you have decided to put it away while treating it, give it some time to breath and apply a gentle but firm scalp massage while encouraging increased stimulation of blood flow.

June · Week of _____

REFLECTION

"A double minded man is unstable in all of his ways" (James 1:8).

I think this is a very bold statement, considering the use of the word *all*. Have you found areas in your life, your thinking, or your relationships that seem to be unstable?

_____

_____

Take time to reflect on your views about the situation and see if it is in agreement with your actions. This could be the deciding factor for what you are able to accomplish.

RESPONSIBILITY

Mon	
Tues	
Wed	
Thu	
Fri	
Sat	
Sun	

REGIMEN: WEEK 2 TYPE

Have you ever noticed that some areas along the same strand may not be consistent? For example, the end of the strand may appear very thin, while the middle is a little thicker, and the hair closest to the root seems to be stronger. As your hair grows longer, it still doesn't have a full effect because the ends allow light to pass through because they are less dense than the hair closer to the root.

This allows you to really see the difference in the type category of a strand. *Type* is the size of the strand and comes in three stages: fine, medium, and course. If measurable, it would be the circumference of the strand. Therefore, you could actually have more than one type along the length of one strand as the cuticle begins to peel its layers due to how the strand is handled.

Hairgistics

Shampoo _____

Conditioner _____

Leave-In _____

Support Product _____

Conditioning time _____

Dryer Time _____ Air dry _____

Protective Style _____

Detangle: Comb _____ Finger _____

Before

Dry	Shedding	Full		
Moist	Breaking	Frizzy		
Oily	Limp	Dull		
Stinky	Heavy	Itchy		
Tangled	Tight	Hard		

After

Dry	Shedding	Full		
Moist	Breaking	Frizzy		
Oily	Limp	Dull		
Stinky	Heavy	Itchy		
Tangled	Tight	Hard		

RELAXATION

Did you know that your heart has a time of relaxation? It's called *cardiac diastole*, and it occurs when the heart relaxes after a contraction. What is most interesting is that it needs this moment of relaxation to prepare for the next refilling of circulating blood. So in order to be refilled, there has to be a relaxation period in the heart so that the body can continue to circulate properly. Thankfully, this is an involuntary muscle, but if it wasn't and it had to depend on you to relax, how long do you think you would be able to survive?

June · Week of _____

REFLECTION

"Forgetting those things which are behind, . . . I press toward the mark for the high calling" (Philippians 3:13-14).

What is your high calling as it relates to your journemony?

_____

_____

Regardless of what you have decided to change, I am sure it is requiring a major transition in your normal routine. The thing I appreciate most about this verse is that it shows the past, present, and future all at the same time. Imagine the wisdom we would have if we saw then what we see now and recognize it at the right time. That would be powerful!

While you are making changes with your hair, you can see through this journal things from the past as you document your process. Simultaneously, you are present every day to participate in the process, and your vision and adjustments support your high calling that you have for your hair. Therefore, release the regrets and lost opportunities, and be conscious that you are making major changes now in the present in order to reach your ultimate vision for your hair.

RESPONSIBILITY

Mon	
Tues	
Wed	
Thu	
Fri	
Sat	
Sun	

REGIMEN: WEEK 3 TRANSITIONING

When considering texture and type of the hair, there could be no better time to really see the difference along the length of the strand. A successful transition involves maintaining as much length as you desire while growing new hair and maintaining your older hair at the same time—trimming only when necessary.

I am currently transitioning from a chemical to natural state, and it's amazing to see the change in texture, type, and density (hairs per square inch) as I allow my hair to obtain length. You will never be able to see the optimum density of the hair until you reclaim your _hairginity_. What does that mean? _Hairginity_ is the purest form of your natural strand, which includes being chemical free, being heat free, using proper detangling methods, and being free of mechanical tools. By allowing this time of rest from unnecessary handling, the strand will experience little to no compromise and can grow to its optimum density and full-length potential.

Hairgistics

Shampoo _____

Conditioner _____

Leave-In _____

Support Product _____

Conditioning time _____

Dryer Time _____ Air dry _____

Protective Style _____

Detangle: Comb _____ Finger _____

Before

Dry	Shedding	Full		
Moist	Breaking	Frizzy		
Oily	Limp	Dull		
Stinky	Heavy	Itchy		
Tangled	Tight	Hard		

After

Dry	Shedding	Full		
Moist	Breaking	Frizzy		
Oily	Limp	Dull		
Stinky	Heavy	Itchy		
Tangled	Tight	Hard		

RELAXATION

Have you ever heard someone say, "Calm your nerves"? Well, based on research, there are some pretty interesting suggestions to consider:

- Give yourself a hand massage.
- Rub your feet over a gold ball.
- Squeeze a stress ball.
- Drip cold water on your wrist and behind your earlobes.
- Wash some dishes.

June · Week of _____

REFLECTION

"And be ye kind one to another, tenderhearted, forgiving one another even as God for Christ's sake hath forgiven you" (Ephesians 4:32).

Although we are a very intelligent creation, we are also very simple—being that we are designed to receive and release, period. If the symphony of your body does not flow properly as instructed, it will malfunction and become imbalanced. Therefore, we must remember for our total health and well-being we must release forgiveness in every opportunity to avoid malfunctioning and becoming stagnant. While you hold the offender to the offense, you are required to be stuck right there with them. Release them so you can move forward.

RESPONSIBILITY

Mon	
Tues	
Wed	
Thu	
Fri	
Sat	
Sun	

REGIMEN: WEEK 4 POROSITY

Porosity is how much or how little moisture your hair will retain based on the disposition of the cuticle. Although the strand looks smooth like a continuous line when stretched out, it's not. The cuticle, as mentioned before, is the outer layer of the strand that protects the other two layers. When magnified, it resembles the roofing shingles on a house: scale-like flaps that should lay flat, one on top of another. However, if there is a breach in the scales, it will affect how much moisture is allowed. When all of the scales are tightly bound, this allows little to no penetration, resulting in hair that is resistant to water or moisture products. This is known as *low porosity*.

If the scales are not as tight and allow for moisture balance, this creates a healthier canvas—a shinier affect with low maintenance, known as *medium porosity*.

Last but not least is *high porosity*. This usually gives off a very frizzy, tangled expression because the cuticles are opened and have too much space to allow too much moisture in and out just as fast.

There is a neat test you can do to determine the porosity of a strand that requires a cup of water and a strand of hair. Place the clean strand in the water and see if the strand stays at the top, middle, or bottom of the cup. The top means low, middle means medium, and bottom means high porosity.

Hairgistics

Shampoo _____

Conditioner _____

Leave-In _____

Support Product _____

Conditioning time _____

Dryer Time _____ Air dry _____

Protective Style _____

Detangle: Comb _____ Finger _____

Before

Dry	Shedding	Full		
Moist	Breaking	Frizzy		
Oily	Limp	Dull		
Stinky	Heavy	Itchy		
Tangled	Tight	Hard		

After

Dry	Shedding	Full		
Moist	Breaking	Frizzy		
Oily	Limp	Dull		
Stinky	Heavy	Itchy		
Tangled	Tight	Hard		

RELAXATION

Have you ever considered that laughing could stimulate circulation and promote muscle relaxation? If not, now you can be more conscious of taking the time to laugh as much as possible during stressful situations. Even if you don't feel like laughing, just do it as a way to trick your body into thinking that it is relaxing in order to receive the positive benefits that it offers.

Journemony Time

Dear Loved One,

Sometimes the hand we are dealt may not be favorable, but always remember . . .

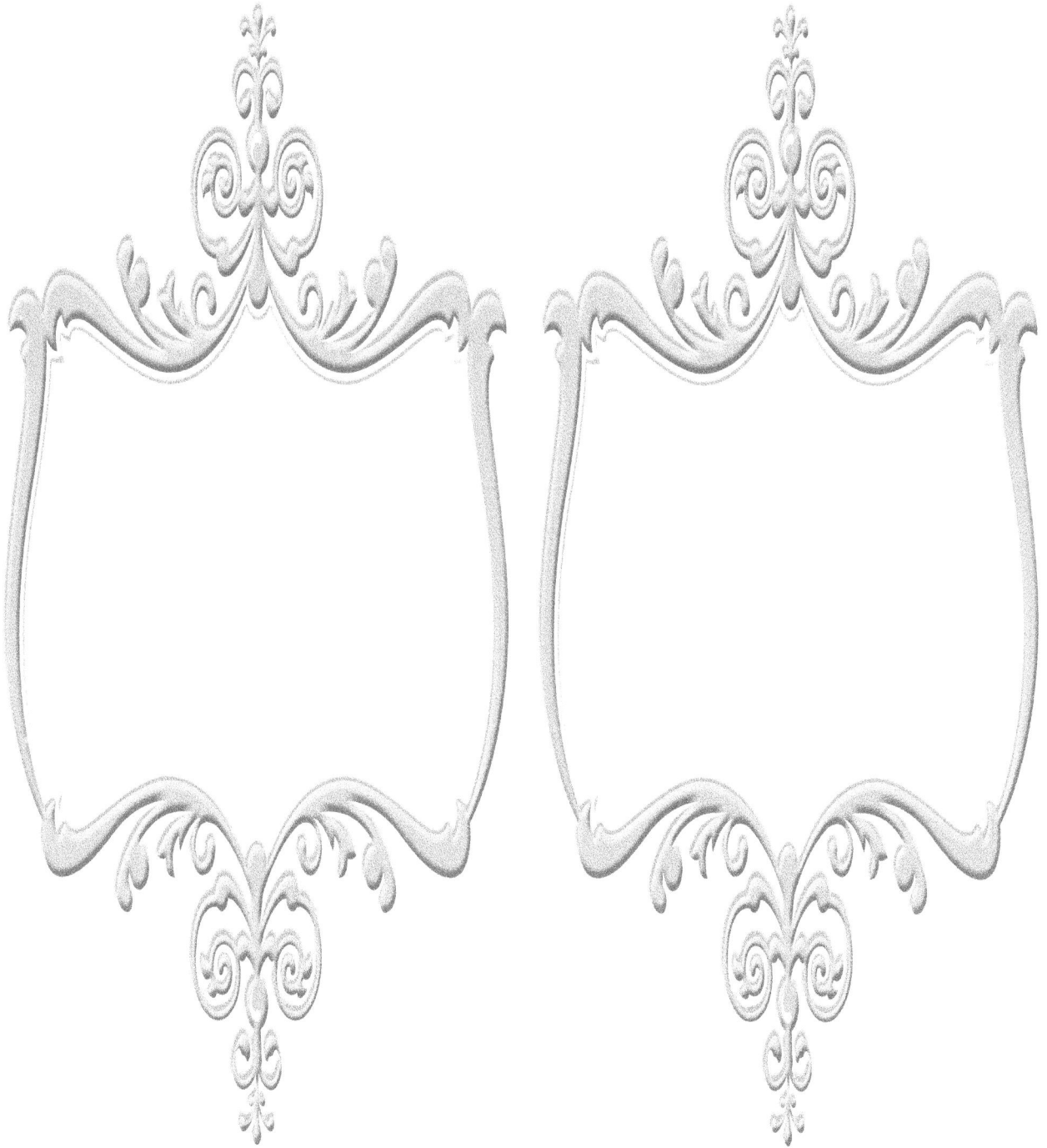

Picture Time

July

Season: Hot & Humid

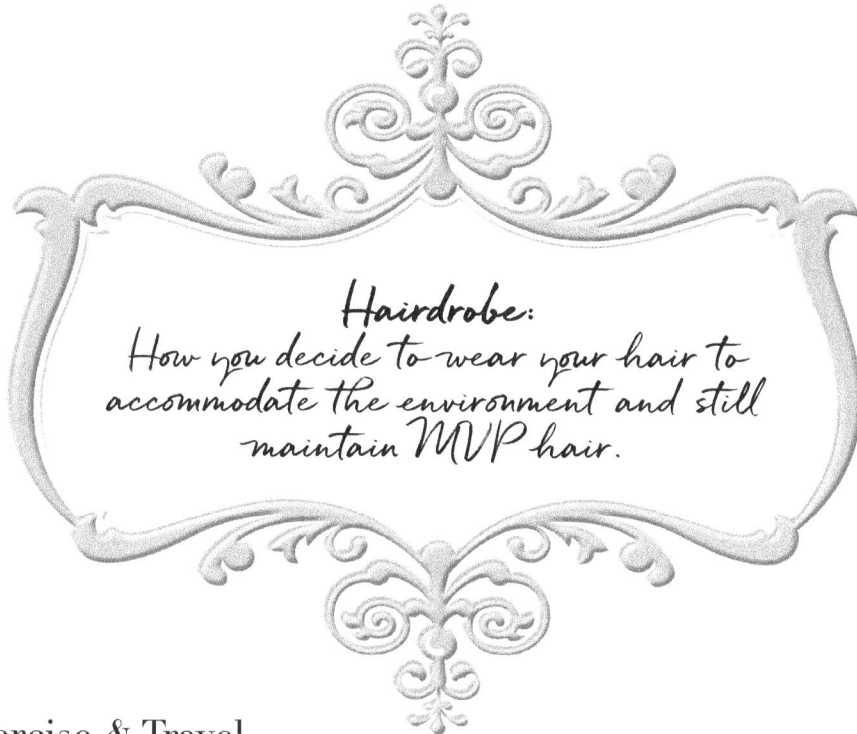

Hairdrobe:
How you decide to wear your hair to accommodate the environment and still maintain MVP hair.

Hairdrobe
Week 1: Exercise & Travel
Week 2: Hairdrobe
Week 3: Swimming
Week 4: Braids

Seasonal Consideration:

Challenge: Keeping the hair and scalp clean

Decision: Quick style options for extra shampoo days

Goal: _____
_____
_____
_____
_____

July · Week of _____

REFLECTION

Did you know that the Bible says that "exercise profited little: but godliness is profitable unto all things"? (1 Timothy 4:8).

I heard someone say, "Although it profits little, I want to benefit from the little that it profits." While I agree, I also believe that this is referring to where your focus is given. For example, you are becoming more aware of your body and getting in shape, while simultaneously neglecting other areas of life that are equally important. Overall, you want to be whole and do those things that profit the whole body, mind, and soul, so you will have balance. If you have an amazing body, but your head is bald, or your mind is negative, you still can't fully enjoy the fruit of your exercise. You will always be in a state of overcompensation for what is off balance.

RESPONSIBILITY

Mon	
Tues	
Wed	
Thu	
Fri	
Sat	
Sun	

REGIMEN: WEEK 1 EXERCISE & TRAVEL

The summer months encourage more exercise and travel. Although this is an exciting time, this is also the time when the schedule changes. Therefore, we must be diligent about remaining on the same schedule as much as possible. Exercising creates more opportunities for excessive sweating, and although this is great for your workout session, it is not as beneficial for your hair. Mind you, I am not just talking about maintaining a style, but maintaining a clean environment for the hair and scalp to flourish.

Just as your body needs to be cleaned daily from regular activity, imagine what it needs when you have sweated in your head during your workout session. Every time you work out and sweat, you can feel the need to shower your body. So why isn't the desire to shampoo the same, considering the hair and scalp have participated in the workout as well? If you have ever shampooed while showering after a workout, you feel even cleaner and more relaxed after the workout. Furthermore, when you sweat, the body will release waste and salt, which automatically causes a drying effect on the hair and scalp, which could ultimately lead to buildup, excessive itching, and an environment for bacteria to cause other scalp disorders. Always shampoo when you sweat in your head during exercise.

Traveling may or may not detour you from your regular schedule; however, it is good to be proactive instead of reactive, especially if you are traveling extensively and have no access to properly condition the hair. I will discuss strategies in the next week to be proactive for exercise and traveling.

Hairgistics

Shampoo _____

Conditioner _____

Leave-In _____

Support Product _____

Conditioning time _____

Dryer Time _____ Air dry _____

Protective Style _____

Detangle: Comb _____ Finger _____

Before

Dry	Shedding	Full		
Moist	Breaking	Frizzy		
Oily	Limp	Dull		
Stinky	Heavy	Itchy		
Tangled	Tight	Hard		

After

Dry	Shedding	Full		
Moist	Breaking	Frizzy		
Oily	Limp	Dull		
Stinky	Heavy	Itchy		
Tangled	Tight	Hard		

RELAXATION

There are all types of techniques and strategies that you can incorporate into your relaxation schedules. There are techniques for sleep, anger, anxiety, pain—and the list goes on and on. However, until the mind has been conditioned to relax, the others are only symptoms that still have a root that needs to be addressed. The immediate gratification may be experienced, but the conflict is sure to resurface if not dealt with at the root. Begin to focus on changing your mind before trying to change how your body responds to your mind.

Hairloom

July · Week of _____

REFLECTION

"Put on the whole armor of God that ye may be able to stand against the wiles of the devil" (Ephesians 6:11).

This verse is all about being prepared for opportunities that may present unforeseen but expected challenges. Any time the adversary is present, you should be proactive instead of reactive. This way, you won't get caught off-guard. As this month may afford you new and exciting opportunities, you may also experience weather and schedule changes in the new environments as you travel. Be sure to think ahead and prepare for any challenges that may hinder the progress of your hair journey.

RESPONSIBILITY

Mon	
Tues	
Wed	
Thu	
Fri	
Sat	
Sun	

REGIMEN: WEEK 2 HAIRDROBES

Traveling takes you out of your normal environment, and based on why you are traveling, may affect how you wear your hair. Therefore, we must be more diligent about not just our wardrobe but also our *hairdrobe*—how you will wear your hair to accommodate the environment and maintain MVP hair.

Time constraints and activity will have the greatest influence on this decision. If you will experience excessive sweating, you will need to shampoo more often and have to have a few quick *hairdrobes*.

While you are packing, consider how you will need to wear your hair as well. Some quick *hairdrobe*s are already set, like braids, that can still be shampooed and thoroughly rinsed and restyled or pulled up. There are also manual "pull back" options that require one or two rollers for a neat bang for frontage appeal. Although it may be hot, I recommend finding a wig, to have more options, and completely keeping the hair as stable as possible until you are back to your normal environment and routine.

Hairgistics

Shampoo _____

Conditioner _____

Leave-In _____

Support Product _____

Conditioning time _____

Dryer Time _____ Air dry _____

Protective Style _____

Detangle: Comb _____ Finger _____

Before

Dry	Shedding	Full		
Moist	Breaking	Frizzy		
Oily	Limp	Dull		
Stinky	Heavy	Itchy		
Tangled	Tight	Hard		

After

Dry	Shedding	Full		
Moist	Breaking	Frizzy		
Oily	Limp	Dull		
Stinky	Heavy	Itchy		
Tangled	Tight	Hard		

RELAXATION

Have you noticed that making changes may also create an environment for unnecessary tension in your life? During this hair journey, please avoid creating unnecessary tension because you are uncomfortable with the way you are wearing your hair. Understand that this is temporary, a means to an end, and will benefit you greatly in the long run. Do not allow the opinion and recommendations of others to form into tension in your life. If you are concerned about how others view your choices and changes in life, you will hinder your vision and focus and produce counterproductive results. Don't allow a source of tension of any kind to stop you. Relax and know that your decisions about your *hairgistics* are the only ones that matter if you are going to succeed and empower the next generation.

July · Week of _____

REFLECTION

"There are, it may be, so many kinds of voices in the world, and none of them is without signification" (1 Corinthians 14:10).

We are created to have amazing ability, and no other individual can stop our progress unless we give them permission. Silence the voices of those that have so much to say but offer no solutions or support. Always be conscious of their motive—not just what you view with your eyes, but also listen for what they are not saying when giving advice. Are they affirming your efforts or just offering *pro-hairbitions*? When you are finished listening, thank them for encouraging you to stay focused. For it is at this time that you will be empowered to become conscious of your progress because it has begun to gain the attention of others.

RESPONSIBILITY

Mon	
Tues	
Wed	
Thu	
Fri	
Sat	
Sun	

REGIMEN: WEEK 3 SWIMMING

Swimming is an excellent activity because the hair is already wet, and there should be no excuse to shampoo after swimming because it is greatly needed. Remember that the cuticle is like the shingles on a roof, except they open and close to allow substances in and out. Therefore, the chlorinated water is allowed in and causes the natural moisture to be removed, leading to a dry environment where breaking and split ends can develop. According to research, it is actually good to take a shower (shampoo and condition the hair) before swimming as well. This has the same effect, as you are preparing the strands and proactively filling the shaft with more product for the chlorine to contend. Although the hair will still be rinsed with the chlorinated water, at least there is a barrier on the strands to rinse instead of nothing at all. So be sure to apply *hairgistics* before and after, especially if you are swimming on a more regular basis. Yes, braids too!

Hairgistics

Shampoo _____

Conditioner _____

Leave-In _____

Support Product _____

Conditioning time _____

Dryer Time _____ Air dry _____

Protective Style _____

Detangle: Comb _____ Finger _____

Before

Dry	Shedding	Full		
Moist	Breaking	Frizzy		
Oily	Limp	Dull		
Stinky	Heavy	Itchy		
Tangled	Tight	Hard		

After

Dry	Shedding	Full		
Moist	Breaking	Frizzy		
Oily	Limp	Dull		
Stinky	Heavy	Itchy		
Tangled	Tight	Hard		

RELAXATION

Relaxation is not just about being still and comfortable. It is actually a state of mind. With consistent practice, you could train your body to relax in any environment. This is the ultimate goal of relaxation techniques: relaxing regardless of your present surroundings. Begin to be mindful of how your body responds in stressful or uncomfortable environments, and refocus your mind to tune in to what is going on within. If you can't seem to calm your body and emotions, it just means that your mind still has capacity to learn how to focus beyond external stimulation.

July · Week of _____

REFLECTION

"But be ye doers of the word, and not hearers only, deceiving your own selves" (James 1:22).

Depending on *where* you start in this journal will affect *how* you start. Thankfully, you are still free to pick what you would like to learn about at your own pace. However, this journal is created for you to be willing and knowledgeable and to apply what is being instructed. If you follow this guide, you will experience things that you could have never imagined about yourself and life in general. Enjoy your journey, and remember that you are taking the next generation with you.

RESPONSIBILITY

Mon	
Tues	
Wed	
Thu	
Fri	
Sat	
Sun	

REGIMEN: WEEK 4 BRAIDS

Braids are the preferred *hairdrobe* for women that are very active—and for children as well. However, braids can be the death of the hair and scalp because it is a convenient and well-set *hairdrobe* that can provide so much versatility. Unfortunately, braids not only create an environment for neglect of the hair and scalp but braids that are too tight also create an environment for hair loss. There is a hairline-loss epidemic throughout the braid population that can result in permanent scar tissue and receding hairlines earlier than expected.

Braids do not have to be tight to be neat. Extra product that has slip should be used at the beginning of every braid, and although it will increase the chances for the hair to be loose, it is better that the hair slip out of the braid than for the hair to be pulled from the root of the scalp. Also, braids should continue to be shampooed and conditioned if planning to wear them longer than a week in order to maintain MVP hair. The last thing you want to do is wear braids and grow some long, weak, porous hair that will not respond to styling because it is so dehydrated. What's the point of growing hair that you can't wear? Even if you have added hair, your hair still needs the same care to flourish. The extensions do not provide a hair-care-free pass just because you don't have to comb it. Your hair is still subject to dirt, dryness, breakage, and everything else it would normally endure if it was worn down.

Hairgistics

Shampoo _____

Conditioner _____

Leave-In _____

Support Product _____

Conditioning time _____

Dryer Time _____ Air dry _____

Protective Style _____

Detangle: Comb _____ Finger _____

Before

Dry	Shedding	Full		
Moist	Breaking	Frizzy		
Oily	Limp	Dull		
Stinky	Heavy	Itchy		
Tangled	Tight	Hard		

After

Dry	Shedding	Full		
Moist	Breaking	Frizzy		
Oily	Limp	Dull		
Stinky	Heavy	Itchy		
Tangled	Tight	Hard		

RELAXATION

You have enough. You do enough. You are enough. Relax.

Journemony Time

Dear Loved One,

As you begin to focus on wholeness and having a healthy lifestyle, always have balance and . . .

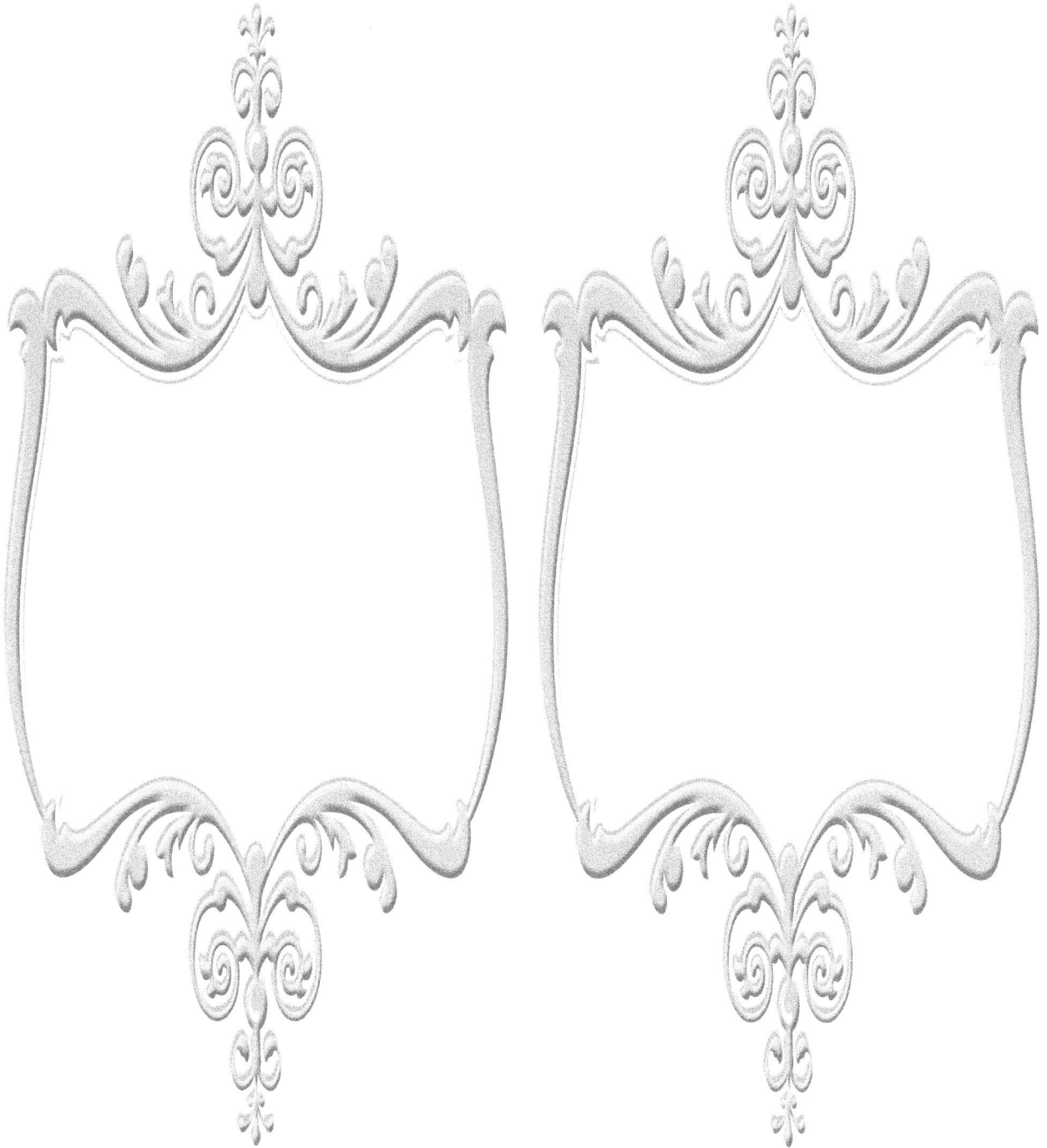

Picture Time

August _____

Season: Hot and Dry

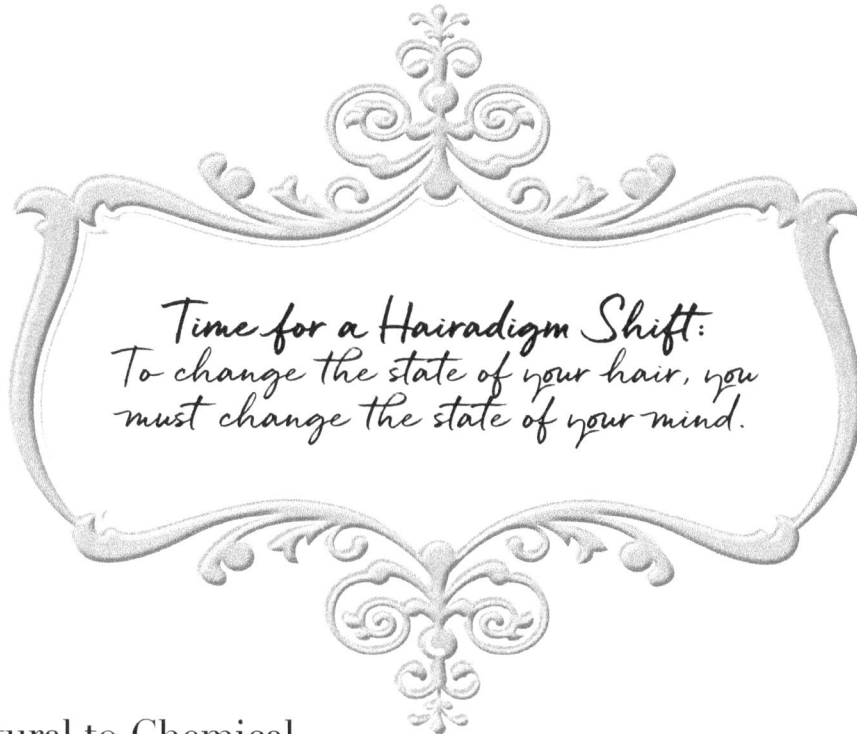

Time for a Hairadigm Shift:
To change the state of your hair, you
must change the state of your mind.

Transitions
Week 1: Natural to Chemical
Week 2: Chemical to Natural
Week 3: Natural to Braids
Week 4: Chemical to Braids

Seasonal Consideration:

Challenge: Keeping the hair and scalp hydrated

Decision: Style choice and hair manipulation

Goal: _____
_____
_____
_____
_____

August · Week of _____

REFLECTION

"And let us not be weary in well doing: for in due to season we shall reap, if we faint not" (Galatians 6:9).

Transitions are always a challenge because it requires change—some that we foresee and some that we never imagined. Either way, change is necessary, and the best way to face a challenge is to declare from the beginning that your perseverance will determine your success. Not how long, how hard, or how strategic you performed in the challenge, but making the decision to not give up until you know that you have done all you can do to change.

RESPONSIBILITY

Mon	
Tues	
Wed	
Thu	
Fri	
Sat	
Sun	

REGIMEN: WEEK 1 NATURAL TO CHEMICAL

Transitions from natural to chemically treated hair can provide you with more smooth style options, but it also requires great attention to conditioning and moisturizing with support products. Some may experience more scalp irritations due to the effects of over drying under hooded dryers as well.

Be sure to continue to maintain *hairgistics* as often as necessary for excessive sweating to ensure a balanced environment for the scalp. Conditioning is key to supply the strands with extra protection for the change in bonds of the cortex of the strand. Anytime the hair is chemically treated, the hair is automatically broken down to a weaker state in order to change the shape of the strand, which allows versatility in styles. During a chemical process, the strands can experience four stages: softening, straightening, thinning, and dissolving. If a chemical relaxer is applied and processed properly, it should only experience the first two stages to have a successful relaxer; anything past that point is creating an environment for breakage and hair loss.

Hairgistics

Shampoo _____

Conditioner _____

Leave-In _____

Support Product _____

Conditioning time _____

Dryer Time _____ Air dry _____

Protective Style _____

Detangle: Comb _____ Finger _____

Before

Dry	Shedding	Full		
Moist	Breaking	Frizzy		
Oily	Limp	Dull		
Stinky	Heavy	Itchy		
Tangled	Tight	Hard		

After

Dry	Shedding	Full		
Moist	Breaking	Frizzy		
Oily	Limp	Dull		
Stinky	Heavy	Itchy		
Tangled	Tight	Hard		

RELAXATION

Did you know that your environment can have a great effect on how you are able to relax? What does your bedroom look like? Is it beautifully decorated with warm cozy decor that invites you to relax? Or is it a big pile of clutter that invites you to clean up? Every space is speaking a specific message. Some spaces pull on the worker in you, while other spaces pull on the relaxation—this is why we like to get away. What would it be like if you could create an environment in your bedroom that is conducive for relaxation?

August · Week of _____

REFLECTION

"For God hath not given us the spirit of fear; but of power, and of love, and of a sound mind" (2 Timothy 1:7).

What do you think causes you fear of meeting challenges?

_____

_____

I believe that a lack of knowledge creates an environment for fear to rule. When we are equipped to face a challenge, all that is left to do is apply what we have learned to apply. Therefore, knowledge and application with determination is a recipe for annihilating fear.

RESPONSIBILITY

Mon	
Tues	
Wed	
Thu	
Fri	
Sat	
Sun	

REGIMEN: WEEK 2 CHEMICAL TO NATURAL

This has become a very popular transition in the last couple of years and is deemed to be a safer and easier way to wear the hair. However, what most fail to realize is that natural hair requires just as much if not more maintenance. Depending on your density, texture, and type, your *hairgistics* can range from low maintenance to requiring a natural hair care professional to step in and save you time that you may not have expected to invest.

If you are transitioning and maintaining your chemically treated hair at the same time, it could become very challenging to avoid breaking the chemically treated hair while simultaneously trying to manage two different types and textures. I definitely recommend a hair care professional if you have over twelve inches of length while trying to transition. It is your decision how much relaxer will be trimmed each month until all of the chemically treated hair is removed. Unfortunately, the chemically treated hair will not revert back to natural after time has passed. Once the bonds in the cortex have been broken and straightened, it is permanent until the hair is cut off.

I recommend *hairdrobes* that will require as little manipulation of the chemically treated hair as possible, as it will be extremely weaker than the new natural hair that is growing from the root. Product choices will also vary based on how you choose to wear your hair. I have had to use setting lotion for one part and natural products for other parts, depending on the style choice. Professional help is greatly recommended for this transition.

Hairgistics

Shampoo _____

Conditioner _____

Leave-In _____

Support Product _____

Conditioning time _____

Dryer Time _____ Air dry _____

Protective Style _____

Detangle: Comb _____ Finger _____

Before

Dry	Shedding	Full		
Moist	Breaking	Frizzy		
Oily	Limp	Dull		
Stinky	Heavy	Itchy		
Tangled	Tight	Hard		

After

Dry	Shedding	Full		
Moist	Breaking	Frizzy		
Oily	Limp	Dull		
Stinky	Heavy	Itchy		
Tangled	Tight	Hard		

RELAXATION

Relaxation starts in the mind. You must learn how to quiet your mind. Sometimes meditation helps, but it is a practice that requires focus and skill over time to really reap the full benefits. Have you ever considered that your mind is full because you need to release what you are holding? There are several ways to do this, but I suggest either recoding it on your phone or writing it out in a journal. That way, you can release everything that is inside of you privately and give your mind time to relax from brainstorming mentally. Brainstorm on paper or digitally until you realize that, if you could fix it, you would have already done it.

August · Week of _____

REFLECTION

"I can do all things through Christ which strengtheneth me" (Philippians 4:13)

What strengthens you? What drives you to move beyond your visible limitations? Do you consider obstacles as a limitation or a motivator to realize your potential?

_____

_____

Be sure that your faith, hope and trust lies in something that is stronger than the greatest version of yourself.

RESPONSIBILITY

Mon	
Tues	
Wed	
Thu	
Fri	
Sat	
Sun	

REGIMEN: WEEK 3 NATURAL TO BRAIDS

As mentioned in the previous month, braids can be very convenient until the hair has been neglected and improperly treated while wearing them. Shampooing and conditioning on top of braids is very possible if you add hair or not. For the sake of the conditioning and moisture level of the hair, it is necessary to treat the hair with the same *hairgistics* to continue the benefits of this journey. I would also recommend creating a leave-in oil spray to keep the braids and scalp as moist as possible during the week.

When you shampoo on top of braids, it is not necessary to ruffle the hair as you shampoo or use a drying towel to rub on top of the braids. Less friction as possible is best. Use a color applicator bottle to apply shampoo in and under the braids, and massage the scalp. Next, be sure to rinse very well until the braids feel squeaky to the touch. Condition with an applicator bottle, also ensuring that the braid is completely saturated. Process under a warm dryer for 15–30 minutes, but check to see if the braid has soaked up the conditioner at the 15-minute mark to determine if more conditioner needs to be added to ensure saturation and deep conditioning. Follow with a thorough rinse and apply the leave-in oil spray to impart moisture and shine.

Of course, the braids will not look as smooth as when they were new, but this is a small price to pay if you decide to keep the braids in longer than a week at a time and still maintain MVP hair.

Hairgistics

Shampoo _____

Conditioner _____

Leave-In _____

Support Product _____

Conditioning time _____

Dryer Time _____ Air dry _____

Protective Style _____

Detangle: Comb _____ Finger _____

Before

Dry	Shedding	Full		
Moist	Breaking	Frizzy		
Oily	Limp	Dull		
Stinky	Heavy	Itchy		
Tangled	Tight	Hard		

After

Dry	Shedding	Full		
Moist	Breaking	Frizzy		
Oily	Limp	Dull		
Stinky	Heavy	Itchy		
Tangled	Tight	Hard		

RELAXATION

Sometimes our own internal dialogue and expectations create tension and unnecessary pressure. Are there any things that you have been holding that you could possibly let go? Imagine that whatever it is that you are holding on to is in your right hand. Now close your hand to conceal it. Hold it as tight as you can, and squeeze until you feel your fingernails in the palm of your hand. Do you feel that tension and sensation? It is not only in your hand but also connected to other parts of your body to maintain that hold. If you were to open your hand and release it, all of the sensation and tension would immediately be relieved. This activity can also be applied to your *hairadigm* and expectations. It is ultimately your choice and free will to make decisions that will be beneficial for your entire well-being. Remember, the truth is the only thing that will set you free.

August · Week of _____

REFLECTION

"In all labour there is profit: but the talk of the lips tendeth only to penury" (Proverbs 14:23).

Life is not going to wait on you to do what you are created to do. It continues as if it never needed you anyway. What others don't know they need will still be an unknown possibility that will continue to have no impact. However, once you set in motion what you have to contribute, there will be an automatic demand that will continue to pull the potential until it becomes possible.

RESPONSIBILITY

Mon	
Tues	
Wed	
Thu	
Fri	
Sat	
Sun	

REGIMEN: WEEK 4 CHEMICAL TO BRAIDS

The same rules of how to handle the braids on a weekly basis applies for this transition as well. However, the weakness of the hair in its chemical state has some other considerations. Be sure to be very careful with the fragility of how tight the braids are applied, especially at the hairline. The strength of the braid with friction could cause tug-of-war hair (more in September) and devastate the condition of your hairline after repeated pulling and friction while styling, sleeping, or braiding. Since the hair is already in a weak state, the heaviness of the braids and excessive styling could cause unnecessary pull on the roots as well. Always remember that the natural hair will always prevail longer than the chemically treated hair, so be extra careful with the stress that is applied on the older, weaker hair.

Hairgistics

Shampoo _____

Conditioner _____

Leave-In _____

Support Product _____

Conditioning time _____

Dryer Time _____ Air dry _____

Protective Style _____

Detangle: Comb _____ Finger _____

Before

Dry	Shedding	Full		
Moist	Breaking	Frizzy		
Oily	Limp	Dull		
Stinky	Heavy	Itchy		
Tangled	Tight	Hard		

After

Dry	Shedding	Full		
Moist	Breaking	Frizzy		
Oily	Limp	Dull		
Stinky	Heavy	Itchy		
Tangled	Tight	Hard		

RELAXATION

Is your mind still racing? Are you worrying? Focusing on something that has not happened—but not in the direction of a favorable outcome—is the perfect recipe for creating unnecessary frustration and depression. Turn the fear into faith, and use the same strategy to expect the best instead of the worst. In other words, relax! And take no thought for tomorrow!

Journemony Time

Dear Loved One,

Sometimes change is necessary and may not be convenient. Always be sure to . . .

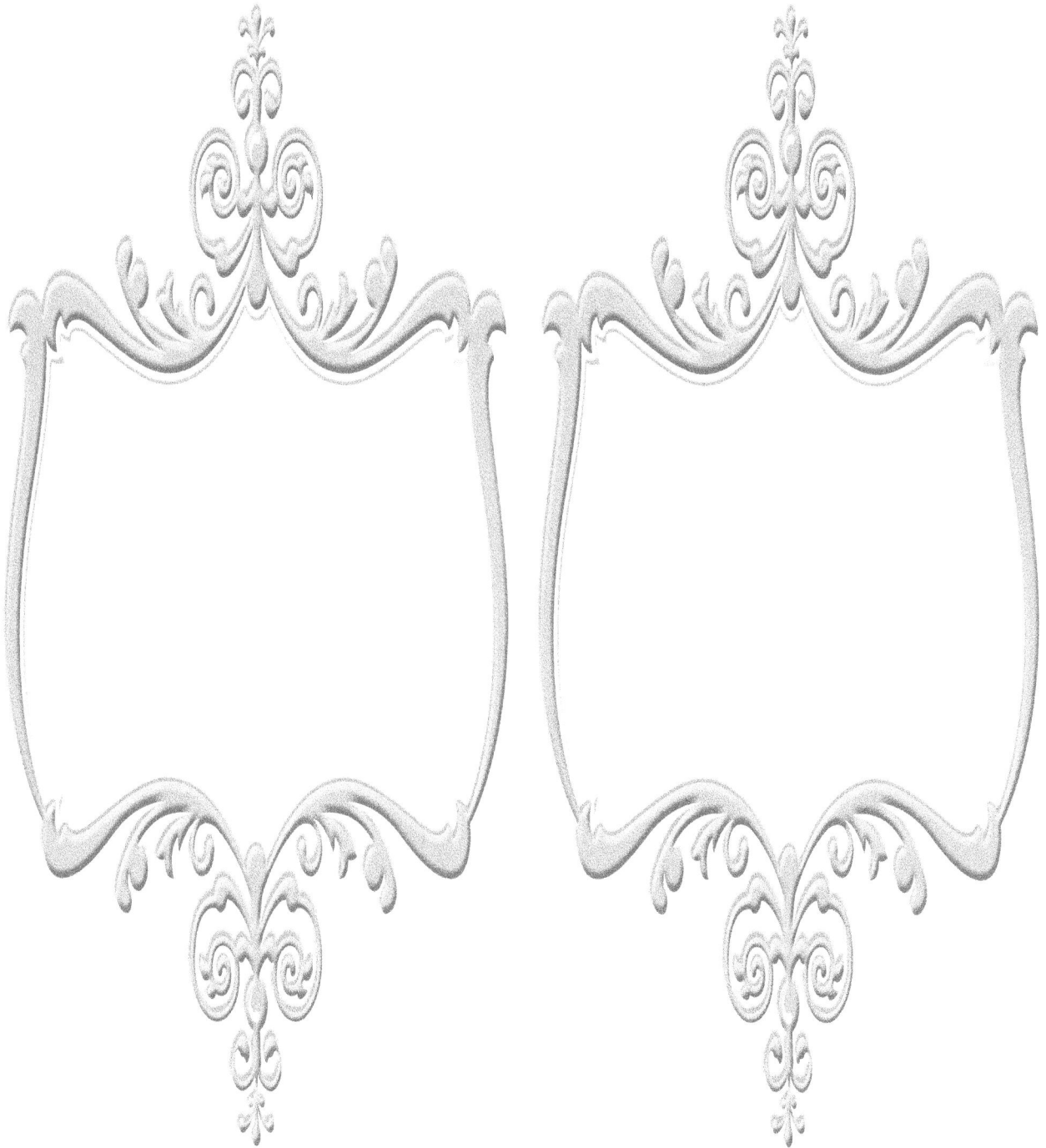

Picture Time

·

September _____

Season: Warm

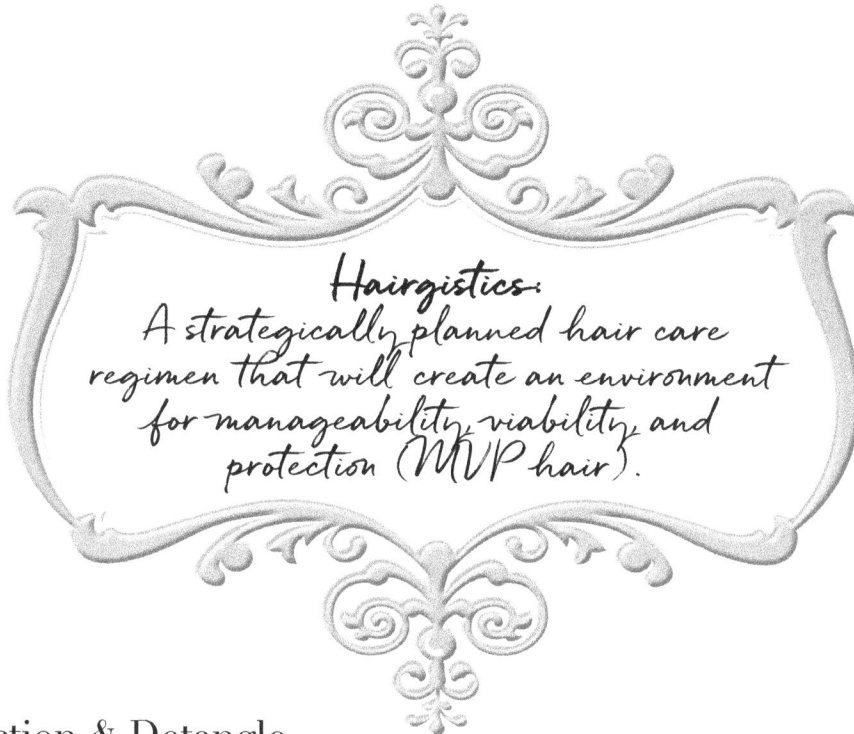

Hairgistics:
A strategically planned hair care regimen that will create an environment for manageability, viability, and protection (MVP hair).

Hairgistics
Week 1: Section & Detangle
Week 2: Shampoo
Week 3: Condition
Week 4: Protect

Seasonal Consideration:

Challenge: Making adjustments based on environment

Decision: Style choice and hair manipulation

Goal: _____
_____
_____
_____
_____

September · Week of _____

REFLECTION

"And beside this, giving all diligence, add to your faith virtue; and to virtue knowledge; and to knowledge temperance; and to temperance patience; and to patience godliness; and to godliness brotherly kindness; and to brotherly kindness charity" (2 Peter 1:5-9).

I may get in trouble with the hair care council, but this verse reminds me of all of the suggestions that bombard the average consumer interested in taking care of their hair. There is always something extra to consider— many choices and varieties of the same product offering different or more advanced results. Unfortunately, you won't truly know unless an extended amount of personal research is applied. This could take a lot of time to experiment and decide what really works. So, allow me to be the voice of reason to break through all of the clutter and confusion in the product selection world: *Truth is anything that stands the test of time without fail, regardless of the circumstances.* I know of only one truth—that's Jesus Christ, the Son of God. Therefore, understand that the only truth you need to know about your hair is that it was created to grow involuntarily, without your help. Ultimately, growth is what is desired. However, how you desire to present and wear your hair is contingent upon what you diligently add to it.

RESPONSIBILITY

Mon	
Tues	
Wed	
Thu	
Fri	
Sat	
Sun	

REGIMEN: WEEK 1 SECTION AND DETANGLE

Before manipulating the hair in any way, sectioning and detangling should be performed. It would be extremely discouraging to lose length and density because of a failed opportunity to take the time to section and detangle the hair before using any type of comb or brush.

Depending on your density and length, sectioning parts will vary. I have found that 4–6 sections will normally prepare the hair for easier detangling sessions. If the hair is not moisturized and more dry than normal, precede the detangling by applying an oil for lubrication and more slip to facilitate the process, avoiding unnecessary breakage. Also, be sure to hold the hair out from the head as you are detangling as opposed to down. I have found that it helps to allow you to see through the hair and determine if shed hair is hindering the fingers from gliding from the root to the ends.

I do not recommend sleeping in rollers; however, there are ways to section the hair based on your style in order to gather the hair in sections that will still accommodate your ability to reproduce the look you are trying to achieve. A roller set can be sectioned off based on the crown, sides, and upper and lower back of the head to individually gather one section at a time. The process of finger combing to remove any shed hairs that may be lingering between curls should be performed to smooth the hair before the support product is applied. Next, creating a curl form that can be safely pinned with a hair pin and covered with a satin cap will ensure a more organized, tangle-free dressing for bed. This way, each section will only have a certain range of movement, discouraging more tangles while friction and moving occurs during bedtime.

Hairgistics

Shampoo _____

Conditioner _____

Leave-In _____

Support Product _____

Conditioning time _____

Dryer Time _____ Air dry _____

Protective Style _____

Detangle: Comb _____ Finger _____

Before

Dry	Shedding	Full		
Moist	Breaking	Frizzy		
Oily	Limp	Dull		
Stinky	Heavy	Itchy		
Tangled	Tight	Hard		

After

Dry	Shedding	Full		
Moist	Breaking	Frizzy		
Oily	Limp	Dull		
Stinky	Heavy	Itchy		
Tangled	Tight	Hard		

RELAXATION

I have come to the conclusion that cleaning is not therapeutic for everyone. However, I have yet to find a person that would not be able to enjoy a clean, organized space if someone else was responsible for the upkeep. You may want to consider finding someone that enjoys cleaning or a housekeeper to help de-clutter your external space while you are creating an environment that is more conducive for relaxation. It will be your relaxation treat.

September · Week of _____

REFLECTION

"Now ye are clean through the word which I have spoken unto you" (John 15:3-5).

As you have probably noticed by now, the section on shampooing is a bit lengthy. I cannot express how important this part of *hairgistics* is to creating an environment for a successful hair journey. Just as we desire clean slates in life due to unfavorable decisions at times, I see shampooing like creating a clean slate to produce different results. Packing new on top of old products will never have the penetration ability that's intended. Therefore, give your hair and the products you are using the proper introduction to determine what combination of products will produce the desired results.

RESPONSIBILITY

Mon	
Tues	
Wed	
Thu	
Fri	
Sat	
Sun	

REGIMEN: WEEK 2 SHAMPOO

Shampoo routines vary from person to person; however, there is a standard that should be considered in order to create MVP hair. The first step is to clean the hair and scalp regularly, whether it is based on your weekly schedule or on an as needed basis. At the very least, you should shampoo every 7 days. Ideal would be every 3 days because that is when the scalp begins to show signs of pollution after the hair has been shampooed. The scalp is responsible for releasing a natural lubricant called *sebum* in order to create an environment that detours bacteria from taking over and causing negative buildup that can lead to a polluted scalp, itching, irritation, and all that makes an uncomfortable environment for the scalp. The hair can also have negative buildup on the shaft level, hindering the cuticle from receiving the conditioning required to create an environment for the smoothing of the cuticle. In order for the hair and scalp to release and receive what it requires, you must have a clean foundation to begin.

A clean environment is conducive to healing because otherwise, bacteria and other germs find a home in polluted environments. It's just the way we are designed. Think about how relieved you feel after the perfect shampoo and massage. It seems to set the stage for all of the other pampering of your spa visit. Next, think about how you feel after sweating profusely and you're not able to shampoo right away. The sweat dries and becomes sticky and stinky. You know you have been around someone whose hair had an odor, or you may have even smelled your own hair at the shampoo bowl during the first rinse. All of that is a response of the hair and scalp when it needs to be cleaned. Please don't neglect the fact that we are designed to be cleaned.

Think of all of the variety of products that are on the market to choose from. However, the hair and scalp require and prefer certain specifications—what is known as the *acid mantle*—that will cause it to flourish over others. The natural pH of the environment that the hair and scalp need to create MVP hair is 4.5–5-5. Without going too far into chemistry, the pH is a range of many substances that lets you know if it is acidic or basic. In this case, the environment of hair is more acidic than basic, which means the products that support the scalp and hair should be close to the same range—otherwise, it will become unbalanced.

An unbalanced environment is a perfect place for disease to flourish. If you decide to ignore the acid-balanced shampoos and you shampoo regularly, your scalp will respond by becoming itchy, flaky, dry, and irritated. Isn't the body amazing how it lets us know its love language? We must not ignore when our hair and scalp are speaking to us because it will give clues to empower us to make necessary *hairgistic* adjustments to support MVP hair.

Hairgistics

Shampoo _____

Conditioner _____

Leave-In _____

Support Product _____

Conditioning time _____

Dryer Time _____ Air dry _____

Protective Style _____

Detangle: Comb _____ Finger _____

Before

Dry	Shedding	Full		
Moist	Breaking	Frizzy		
Oily	Limp	Dull		
Stinky	Heavy	Itchy		
Tangled	Tight	Hard		

After

Dry	Shedding	Full		
Moist	Breaking	Frizzy		
Oily	Limp	Dull		
Stinky	Heavy	Itchy		
Tangled	Tight	Hard		

RELAXATION

Sometimes a person's bedroom is not fully conducive for relaxing. Do you have a TV in your room? This sends a message of entertainment, not relaxation. And yes, there is a difference. Depending on the content, you could be causing your mind and body unnecessary tension and stress. Pay more attention to how a show makes you feel because it could be programming your nervous system to respond to other things in life that's not beneficial to your health—and not even real.

September · Week of _____

REFLECTION

"Come unto me, all ye that labour and are heavy laden, and I will give you rest" (Matthew 11:28).

Sometimes the best way to rest is to release and delegate to someone else. What have you taken on that could be handled by someone that you trust?

_____

_____

Is it really necessary to be the hero in every area of everyone's life? Imagine how much more empowered you would be if you empowered someone else to rise to the occasion and lend a helping hand. We must strengthen the next generation so there will be a firm foundation to continue building.

RESPONSIBILITY

Mon	
Tues	
Wed	
Thu	
Fri	
Sat	
Sun	

REGIMEN: WEEK 3 CONDITION

The conditioning process is not for the purpose of making your hair healthy. Conditioning is a process used to create a softer more manageable environment to produce desired results. Therefore, conditioning will not help the hair to grow (ask anyone that wears dreadlocks). Just like a workout is a type of conditioning, it does not, in and of itself, change the body immediately or cause the body to be healthy. It is only one part of a combination of things that will support the desired result of health, flexibility, and energy.

Healthy hair is determined at the root of the strand. And how you handle it as it emerges and grows will indicate if the hair is responding to your efforts. Since you can't actually see the root of the strand, the viability of the shaft has to be determined by its presence. If there is a visible strand, there is hope. However, as the strand continues to grow, *hairgistics* must be applied to support MVP hair.

Everything concerning the physiology of the body requires information or stimulation to be given and received. When the body receives something, it is designed to process the information and produce a response. Therefore, the scalp and hair are the same. When the scalp receives a shampoo, conditioner, or massage, it will produce the proper environment that encourages MVP hair.

Proper stimulation provides information for the inner working of the dermis to respond with necessary blood flow to the follicle. Life is in the blood, and this is why a strand test can identify the substances like medications, drugs, etc., that have been introduced to the body. Stimulation can also help to relieve tension by encouraging blood flow to an area of the scalp. Be sure to lubricate the scalp before a massage to avoid unnecessary friction on otherwise dryer areas of the hair. The best stimulation can be experienced while shampooing, as the scalp and hair are already moist and lubricated with shampoo, and the fingers have more mobility to glide across the scalp and provide relief and stimulation.

Hairgistics

Shampoo _____

Conditioner _____

Leave-In _____

Support Product _____

Conditioning time _____

Dryer Time _____ Air dry _____

Protective Style _____

Detangle: Comb _____ Finger _____

Before

Dry	Shedding	Full		
Moist	Breaking	Frizzy		
Oily	Limp	Dull		
Stinky	Heavy	Itchy		
Tangled	Tight	Hard		

After

Dry	Shedding	Full		
Moist	Breaking	Frizzy		
Oily	Limp	Dull		
Stinky	Heavy	Itchy		
Tangled	Tight	Hard		

RELAXATION

I pray that requiring more knowledge about how to take care of your hair relieves you of unnecessary anxiety with your *hairloom*. You can relax knowing that as long as you see a strand peeking through the scalp, no matter how small, there is a source of life beneath that is created to produce a hair. Less stress and anxiety will free your blood flow to have balance and proper cardiac rhythm, which will greatly influence the heart of your hair to stimulate follicular activity conducive for growth.

September · Week of _____

REFLECTION

"But whosoever drinketh of the water that I shall give him shall never thirst; but the water that I shall give him shall be in him a well of water springing up into everlasting life" (John 4:14).

Not only are we responsible for external hydration but also internal hydration. What are you filled with that causes you to flow and operate at your optimum state? Are you only hydrating yourself with yourself?

_____

_____

That would lead to extreme dehydration and ultimately disease, whether mental or physical. Consider being renewed in the spirit of your mind by opening up to the only powerful source that saw fit to create you in the first place.

RESPONSIBILITY

Mon	
Tues	
Wed	
Thu	
Fri	
Sat	
Sun	

REGIMEN: WEEK 4 PROTECT

When it comes to overall protection of the hair, it depends on what you desire for your hair to do. Normally we desire for the hair to have optimum density and length to support a desired style and manageability. With these desires in mind, we need to apply *hairgistics* based on our individual expectations. Therefore, we want to provide protection from losing hair prematurely and from any products that will cause the hair to be dry and unmanageable. As discussed in week 2 of January, every style decision should provide a foundation of protection for the overall manageability and vitality of the hair and scalp.

A hydrated environment is necessary to avoid dryness, irritation, and potential breakage. Many things can cause a dry environment, which includes what you receive and expose your hair and scalp to. One method to proactively hydrate the scalp is to understand the difference between the use of moisture products and oil. Moisture is to hydrate an area, while the oil does not hydrate but rather helps to seal the hydration that has been applied.

Your scalp has a natural lubrication but not enough to fight the internal and external environment that contends with it. Therefore, you must apply oil—one that will not clog the pores—to the hydrated scalp after rinsing conditioner and before continuing with the other products and style process. Always protect the scalp with oil before sitting under a hooded dryer, especially in the crown area that endures the most direct heat of any other part of the head.

The hair should be treated in the same manner; protect the shaft with oil or a heat protectant product to coat the cuticle of the strand. Oil should not be used as the hydration product; it can only seal the previous condition of the environment. This is why you can apply oil to a dirty scalp and it still itches. You have only successfully sealed in the dirty, itchy condition that was already present. This reinforces the importance of beginning with a clean environment before applying product.

Hairgistics

Shampoo _____

Conditioner _____

Leave-In _____

Support Product _____

Conditioning time _____

Dryer Time _____ Air dry _____

Protective Style _____

Detangle: Comb _____ Finger _____

Before

Dry	Shedding	Full		
Moist	Breaking	Frizzy		
Oily	Limp	Dull		
Stinky	Heavy	Itchy		
Tangled	Tight	Hard		

After

Dry	Shedding	Full		
Moist	Breaking	Frizzy		
Oily	Limp	Dull		
Stinky	Heavy	Itchy		
Tangled	Tight	Hard		

RELAXATION

When was the last time you sat in a comfortable and quiet place with *no* distractions? Don't you think you deserve to treat yourself to some "me" time?

Journemony Time

Dear Loved One,

Anything that you are going to attempt to excel in will require . . .

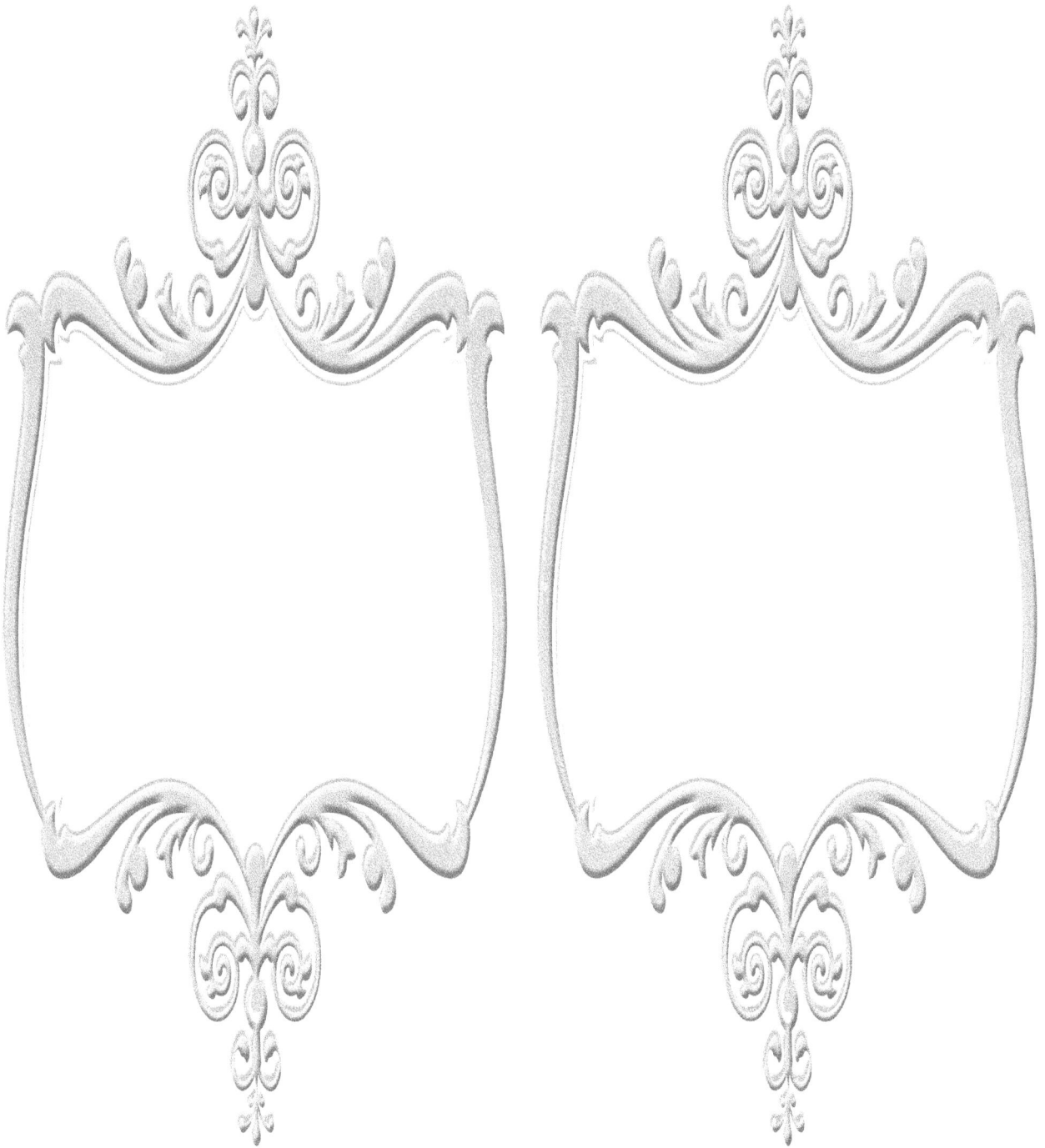

Picture Time

October _____

Season: Cool

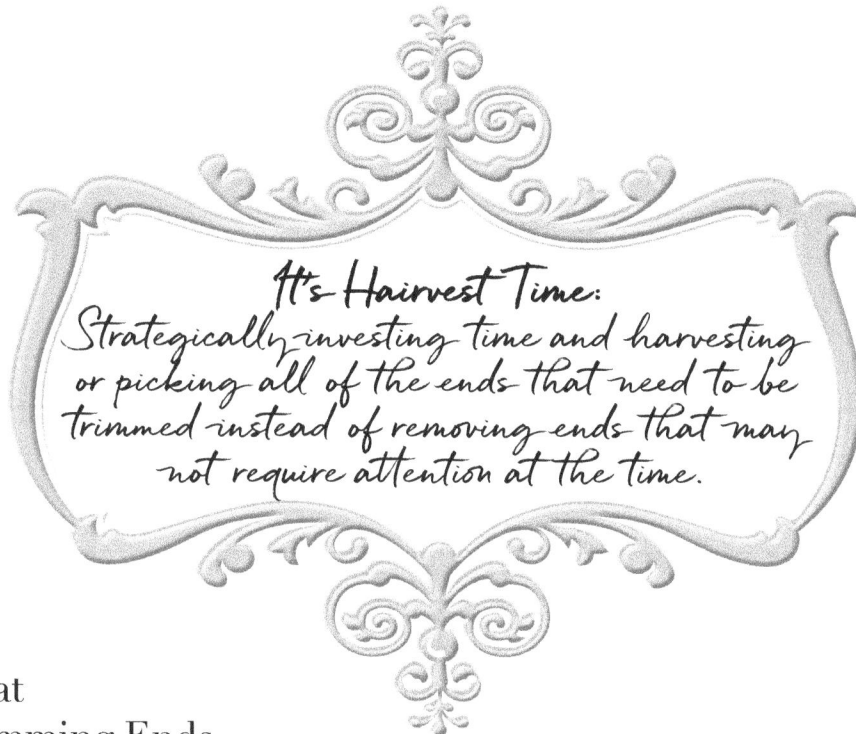

It's Hairvest Time:
Strategically investing time and harvesting
or picking all of the ends that need to be
trimmed instead of removing ends that may
not require attention at the time.

Trim or Treat
Week 1: Trimming Ends
Week 2: Treating Ends
Week 3: Strand Integrity
Week 4: Strand Protection

Seasonal Consideration:

Challenge: Keeping the hair and scalp hydrated

Decision: Style choice and hair manipulation

Goal: _____
_____
_____
_____
_____

October · Week of _____

REFLECTION

"Study to show thyself approved unto God, a workman that needeth not to be ashamed, rightly dividing the word of truth" (2 Timothy 2:15).

Anything that is important to your well-being and life in general should be studied. Avoid being lazy when it comes to learning something new or obtaining information necessary to do your very best. A lot of your life has been spent in school. You have possibly invested money in higher education, and it provided an environment for you to study to become more confident and knowledgeable about how to operate. Remember, the body is designed to receive, process, and release a response to continue performing at its very best. Pay attention to your hair and anything else that means something to you, and begin to research how to take care of your life beyond what you see or hear from others. Go beyond the status quo and become responsible for your progress.

RESPONSIBILITY

Mon	
Tues	
Wed	
Thu	
Fri	
Sat	
Sun	

REGIMEN: WEEK 1 TRIMMING ENDS

Ends are very important when it comes to length retention and optimal fullness. The condition that the ends are in can make or break a style, whether short or long. Ends help to give the hair the weight it needs to hold a curl properly and provide movement. Without the optimum fullness of the ends, a style can literally become a flop. The tricky thing about ends is that all of them are not at the end of the majority of the length of the hair. This is due in part to how the hair grows in cycles and how the strand is conditioned and handled on a daily basis. Since each strand is subject to different lengths, there is no way to completely trim all of the ends by cutting off the ends of the length of the hair. This is why trimming should be done on an as-needed basis; just because you trim the ends of the majority of the length doesn't mean you have addressed all of the ends that may need to be trimmed.

Furthermore, the likelihood of every end needing to be trimmed is slim to none. This is a good reason to be more proactive with your ends than reactive. There are a few terms and strategies used for trimming ends; however, I prefer to call it *hairvesting* the ends. *Hairvesting* the ends, although time consuming, will ensure you address the entire head. This will require sectioning the hair and holding individual subsections at a 90-degree angle from the head until you have trimmed all of the ends that need attention. This way, you are strategically investing time and harvesting or picking all of the ends that need to be trimmed instead of removing ends that may not require attention at the time.

Hairgistics

Shampoo _____

Conditioner _____

Leave-In _____

Support Product _____

Conditioning time _____

Dryer Time _____ Air dry _____

Protective Style _____

Detangle: Comb _____ Finger _____

Before

Dry	Shedding	Full		
Moist	Breaking	Frizzy		
Oily	Limp	Dull		
Stinky	Heavy	Itchy		
Tangled	Tight	Hard		

After

Dry	Shedding	Full		
Moist	Breaking	Frizzy		
Oily	Limp	Dull		
Stinky	Heavy	Itchy		
Tangled	Tight	Hard		

RELAXATION

Did you know that you can create relaxing environments anywhere you go? Even at work, the grocery store, or school. Just as you associate certain external sounds and activities with relaxation, you can reproduce some of those environments in other places. That way, you can remain in a conscious state of relaxation more often than not. Depending on your environment, you may only be able to use headphones to listen to some relaxing music or light your favorite candle in your office space. How about removing your shoes under your desk and propping them on a soft microform pillow? Anything that will soften your experience can be an idea to relax the body.

October · Week of _____

REFLECTION

Did you know that you are the steward of your life? God is the owner and Creator, but you are the steward or manager. You have been given dominion over all things pertaining to life and godliness. Do not allow your present circumstance to trick you into a victim mentality state of being. You are more powerful than you know. Begin to find out about your Creator and how He intended for you to operate so you can discontinue operating in a malfunctioning state due to a lack of knowledge. Ask God to show you His purpose for your life.

RESPONSIBILITY

Mon	
Tues	
Wed	
Thu	
Fri	
Sat	
Sun	

REGIMEN: WEEK 2 TREATING ENDS

Since the ends are the oldest part of the strand, it has experienced more wear and tear than the shaft and roots. Also, it is normally the more dehydrated part because it is the part farthest away from the natural sebum that is provided by the scalp. Depending on the length, even daily brushing would not allow the sebum to ever reach the ends, depending on the length. Therefore, it is our responsibility to use support products to keep the shaft and ends of the strand moisturized and sealed.

Unfortunately, there is no such thing as a product that can repair your ends; therefore, the ends have to be treated in order for you to hold on to it until you are ready to *hairvest* the ends. The repair treatments are used for sealing the ends with a product that will help to flatten the cuticle and lubricate the ends to avoid more dehydration. Moisturized and sealed ends will help avoid splitting.

However, damage that results from the cortical fibers due to chemical processing is another story. When the fibers are unraveled from the inside out, potential damage is inevitable to affect any part of the strand at any time. The treatment will require extensive care and time until a new cycle of hair releases that strand from duty.

Hairgistics

Shampoo _____

Conditioner _____

Leave-In _____

Support Product _____

Conditioning time _____

Dryer Time _____ Air dry _____

Protective Style _____

Detangle: Comb _____ Finger _____

Before

Dry	Shedding	Full		
Moist	Breaking	Frizzy		
Oily	Limp	Dull		
Stinky	Heavy	Itchy		
Tangled	Tight	Hard		

After

Dry	Shedding	Full		
Moist	Breaking	Frizzy		
Oily	Limp	Dull		
Stinky	Heavy	Itchy		
Tangled	Tight	Hard		

RELAXATION

The greatest source of relaxation comes from within, when we are able to settle and quiet our minds from self-talk. Unfortunately, because we are normally so busy and do not take the time to proactively prioritize and plan our daily activities, the mind has to become a sort of personal assistant to keep track of all the possible things that you could encounter.

Relaxing yourself involves bringing balance to your schedule and process. Write your to-do list for the next day before bed, and determine that anything that is not a life or death situation will have to wait until you plan it, if it is not on the list that you already set. This should create for more balance and less tension from the unknown when we schedule and prioritize our daily activities.

October · Week of _____

REFLECTION

"Therefore, my beloved brethren, be ye steadfast, unmovable, always abounding in the work of the Lord, forasmuch as ye know that your labor is not in vain in the Lord" (1 Corinthians 15:58).

Otherwise known as, "Only what you do for Christ will last." This is a good motive tester. Does your motivation to help and encourage come from how a person treats you or from a place of need? What happens when what you perceive to be needed is not appreciated? Do you persist?

_____

_____

This is a very sensitive issue, because according to our Creator, we should respond to challenges based on His grace and not on our own ability and convenience. Check your motive and make sure that you are responding to God's request before responding to a situation that you have not been assigned.

RESPONSIBILITY

Mon	
Tues	
Wed	
Thu	
Fri	
Sat	
Sun	

REGIMEN: WEEK 3 STRAND INTEGRITY

Strand integrity is when the strands are compact—meaning the cuticle scales are laid down and there is no internal damage to the cortical fibers of the strand that will prevent the cuticle from fully protecting the inside. The integrity of the strand produces strength, elasticity, and a smooth appearance that reflects light and shine. When the cuticle or outer layer of the shaft is compromised, the porosity will shift based on the external environment of the strand and will determine the strand's ability to receive and release products. Determining *hairgistics* suitable for your individual needs, whether natural or chemically treated, will help to maintain the integrity of the shaft.

Hairgistics

Shampoo _____

Conditioner _____

Leave-In _____

Support Product _____

Conditioning time _____

Dryer Time _____ Air dry _____

Protective Style _____

Detangle: Comb _____ Finger _____

Before

Dry	Shedding	Full		
Moist	Breaking	Frizzy		
Oily	Limp	Dull		
Stinky	Heavy	Itchy		
Tangled	Tight	Hard		

After

Dry	Shedding	Full		
Moist	Breaking	Frizzy		
Oily	Limp	Dull		
Stinky	Heavy	Itchy		
Tangled	Tight	Hard		

RELAXATION

Have you considered going to the gym and working out for a few minutes to experience the relaxation of the steam room or hot tub? Also, swimming or soaking may be another relaxing activity to consider.

October · Week of _____

REFLECTION

Is your love free?

_____

_____

When we decide to do things that affect other people, we must be aware of the motivation behind our response. Sometimes, a lot of our conflict comes because our motive is not conducive for our capacity to love freely. If you have conflict in relationships due to a difference of opinion, it should not affect the regard you have for that individual. It should, however, cause you to look within to see what is motivating your response. If love according to the Creator is not your motivation, then you must consider refocusing your attention toward being reconciled rather than being right.

RESPONSIBILITY

Mon	
Tues	
Wed	
Thu	
Fri	
Sat	
Sun	

REGIMEN: WEEK 4 STRAND PROTECTION

The strand has so many opportunities to be harmed that it is a challenge to have a completely damage-free environment when wearing your hair.

This is why it is important to allow for careful attention to the strand from root to tip during the maintenance of the hair. Reclaiming your *hairginity* is a good way to avoid unnecessary tension on the strand. The careful use of your hands and fingers with products that support the natural needs of the strand establishes proper *hairgistics*. Protection from environmental pollutants and drying products will contribute to the protection of the strand.

As you can see by now, this journal is about the manageability, viability, and protection of the hair and scalp at all cost. Wearing a style should always be dependent upon how you desire to protect your strands, not the other way around.

Hairgistics

Shampoo _____

Conditioner _____

Leave-In _____

Support Product _____

Conditioning time _____

Dryer Time _____ Air dry _____

Protective Style _____

Detangle: Comb _____ Finger _____

Before

Dry	Shedding	Full		
Moist	Breaking	Frizzy		
Oily	Limp	Dull		
Stinky	Heavy	Itchy		
Tangled	Tight	Hard		

After

Dry	Shedding	Full		
Moist	Breaking	Frizzy		
Oily	Limp	Dull		
Stinky	Heavy	Itchy		
Tangled	Tight	Hard		

RELAXATION

Time for a getaway. Do you or someone else you know like to drive? Sometimes a drive through beautiful scenery can take you to a place of relaxation—to get away from the familiar sights, sounds, and activities of your normal routine.

Journemony Time

Dear Loved One,

No one can be you; by the same token, you cannot be anyone else. Make sure
you are . . .

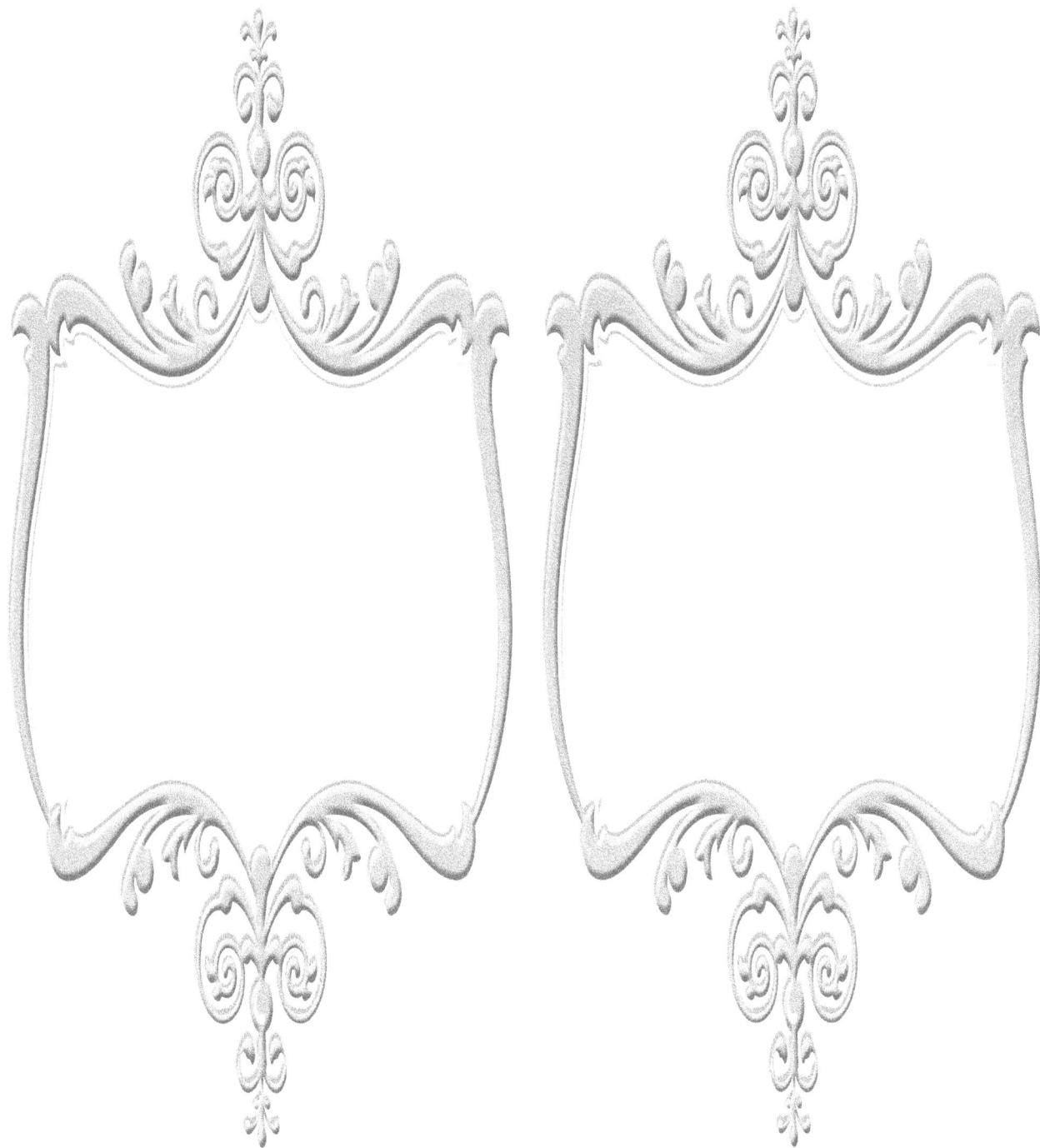

Picture Time

November _____

Season: Cool to Cold

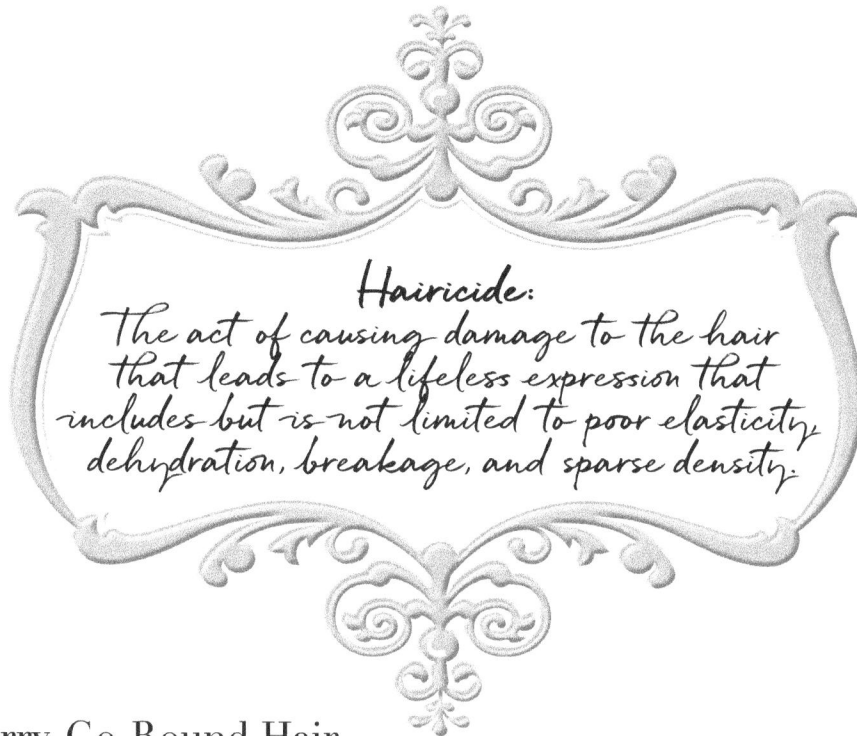

Hairicide:
The act of causing damage to the hair that leads to a lifeless expression that includes but is not limited to poor elasticity, dehydration, breakage, and sparse density.

Hairicide
Week 1: Merry-Go-Round Hair
Week 2: Peek-a-Boo Hair
Week 3: You Are So Sensitive, Scalp
Week 4: Tug-of-War Hair

Seasonal Consideration:

Challenge: Hairgistics for MVP hair

Decision: Style choice and hair manipulation

Goal: _____
_____
_____
_____
_____

November · Week of _____

REFLECTION

"Through faith, we understand that the worlds were framed by the word of God, so that things which are seen were not made of things which do appear" (Hebrews 11:3).

In other words, what you see is not what you get. Consider a cake: it's a fluffy, (hopefully) moist sponge-like material that has flavor and fragrance to please the palette. However, the ingredients used to make the cake may not be as pleasing if devoured individually. If eaten separately, you would not be able to even come remotely close to tasting the end result of the cake you are trying to produce. They must all first come together to make the end product. Same applies to other things in life— challenges or opportunities are just ingredients that come together to produce that final victory that will be pleasing to your purpose. Stay focused and allow all of the ingredients to come together and be properly baked before turning off the heat.

RESPONSIBILITY

Mon	
Tues	
Wed	
Thu	
Fri	
Sat	
Sun	

REGIMEN: WEEK 1 MERRY-GO-ROUND HAIR

Although a merry-go-round can be fun and relaxing, at some point, you will realize that although you are moving, there is no progression. Year after year, many accept the same results from their *hairgistics* without requiring progress. This should be unacceptable, knowing that hair and scalp care will respond differently when given different *hairgistics*.

The beauty of trichology is in the detailed observation of the strand and scalp via handheld microscopes. This allows a more concrete diagnosis of the cause of hair and scalp disorders. Without a microscopic view, you could focus on addressing more superficial issues while overlooking root causes of hair issues. Microscopically, you will find issues that contribute to poor elasticity, chronic split ends, and porosity, as well as texture and type changes, in the manifestation of layer peeling, tears, and bubbles in the hair strands—and in some cases, slight color changes due to extreme dehydration.

Hairgistics

Shampoo _____

Conditioner _____

Leave-In _____

Support Product _____

Conditioning time _____

Dryer Time _____ Air dry _____

Protective Style _____

Detangle: Comb _____ Finger _____

Before

Dry	Shedding	Full		
Moist	Breaking	Frizzy		
Oily	Limp	Dull		
Stinky	Heavy	Itchy		
Tangled	Tight	Hard		

After

Dry	Shedding	Full		
Moist	Breaking	Frizzy		
Oily	Limp	Dull		
Stinky	Heavy	Itchy		
Tangled	Tight	Hard		

RELAXATION

How to relax in traffic? I have found that if I schedule to leave an hour before the time of my next destination, I immediately take the pressure of time constrains off of my trip. It also gives me time to be early and take a moment to get myself together and fully focus on my next assignment, since I will most likely be early for the next appointment. Try it and see if it works for you. This is a good way to be proactive in living a relaxed life.

November · Week of _____

REFLECTION

"Preach the word, be instant in season and out of season" (2 Timothy 4:2).

Although this scripture is referring to spreading the gospel of Jesus Christ, it can also be used as a principle for any situation, whether we think it is time or not. Anything that is important to you that is worthy of respect should have your attention and be a part of what you share in your message of life—better known as your *testimony*. Be prepared to give an answer, especially in this information age. There should be no reason for ignorance when there are several opportunities to research a variety of sources on a subject that is important to your life. I personally suggest study of the Word of God—it has all of the answers you could ever need for every season of life.

RESPONSIBILITY

Mon	
Tues	
Wed	
Thu	
Fri	
Sat	
Sun	

REGIMEN: WEEK 2 PEEK-A-BOO HAIR

As previously stated, what you see is not what you get. Although not very common, you may find that an area that appears to be balding or thinning, presenting itself as alopecia, may be a more superficial issue that originates not from the blood but from the surface of the epidermis or scalp. Sometimes the hair can be blocked in the mouth of the follicle (the pore where the hair emerges). This can appear as balding if the condition becomes chronic. Or the hairs can be very short and subject to continued stress, so it cannot obtain or retain length due to improper *hairgistics*. Unfortunately, the way to identify this is with the aid of a handheld microscope, so you would need to consult a trichologist for this concern.

Hairgistics

Shampoo _____

Conditioner _____

Leave-In _____

Support Product _____

Conditioning time _____

Dryer Time _____ Air dry _____

Protective Style _____

Detangle: Comb _____ Finger _____

Before

Dry	Shedding	Full		
Moist	Breaking	Frizzy		
Oily	Limp	Dull		
Stinky	Heavy	Itchy		
Tangled	Tight	Hard		

After

Dry	Shedding	Full		
Moist	Breaking	Frizzy		
Oily	Limp	Dull		
Stinky	Heavy	Itchy		
Tangled	Tight	Hard		

RELAXATION

Sometimes just a little knowledge about something can put you in a relaxed state. For example, if you were warned that a tornado was predicted within the next twenty-four hours, this would give you an opportunity to prepare before it hits. While others that were not prepared may be running around frantic, trying to prepare and take cover, you would have already had the opportunity because of a little knowledge to prepare within a less stressful environment. Therefore, your knowledge would create a more relaxed state during what could have been a very tense situation. Stay knowledgeable and prepared concerning things that have otherwise created stress or tension in your life.

November · Week of _____

REFLECTION

"Where there is no vision, the people perish: but he that keepeth the law, happy is he" (Proverbs 29:18).

Have you ever set a vision for your own life, or are you allowing life to set it for you?

_____

_____

Setting a vision provides a focus for you to stay on track as you pursue your desires. A vision is a reminder of what you expect to accomplish in your life. Without a focus, the path you take will not be stable. Without stability, the direction you need to follow will not be clear, possibly leading to an undesirable end.

RESPONSIBILITY

Mon	
Tues	
Wed	
Thu	
Fri	
Sat	
Sun	

REGIMEN: WEEK 3 YOU ARE SO SENSITIVE, SCALP

An environment of the epidermis (scalp) that produces a chronic itch, excessive shedding, redness, irritation, and inflammation of any kind is indicative of a sensitive scalp. The reason for labeling it as sensitive is because the symptoms are subjective to each individual.

Now, I realize that symptoms bring awareness to the body to indicate that something is not balanced. However, what we want to avoid is creating more symptoms based on a lack of knowledge and a wild imagination.

What I love the most about a diagnosis is when the doctors say that the cause is not known and can vary based on several different factors. Here is where the playground gets crowded, and it's time to step back to see what is really going on. If there are symptoms, it means something else is going on that you cannot see. Therefore, since you or the doctor cannot see the origination of the symptoms, you can determine whatever you want to receive as the cause. Hence, for this disorder, or imbalance, we are going to determine that the cause is a lack of creating proper *hairgistics* for the hair and scalp. By implementing what the skin originally requires, balance and healing should follow based on how the skin works, disallowing the disorder to remain. I have personally seen this disorder completely vanish with application of *hairgistics*, so let this be your starting point to a balanced, healthy environment.

Hairgistics

Shampoo _____

Conditioner _____

Leave-In _____

Support Product _____

Conditioning time _____

Dryer Time _____ Air dry _____

Protective Style _____

Detangle: Comb _____ Finger _____

Before

Dry	Shedding	Full		
Moist	Breaking	Frizzy		
Oily	Limp	Dull		
Stinky	Heavy	Itchy		
Tangled	Tight	Hard		

After

Dry	Shedding	Full		
Moist	Breaking	Frizzy		
Oily	Limp	Dull		
Stinky	Heavy	Itchy		
Tangled	Tight	Hard		

RELAXATION

How to relax during grocery shopping? If you have to make a trip, since we have all of this new technology and curbside service available, make sure it is during a time where there is less traffic—like during the early morning hours. Or map out your list with the flow of your store of choice, and strategically travel down each aisle as you listen with earphones to your own relaxing music. At all cost, if at all possible, do not travel with anyone that may cause unnecessary pressure or stress during this event. Also, consider making a monthly shopping list so that you can take as few trips as possible. This would further cut down on the opportunity for grocery shopping stress. If none of these suggestions work for you, you must determine in your mind that the feeling of stress during grocery shopping is just a reminder of past anxiety. Therefore, each trip is a new opportunity to create a new experience that will not allow stress to take the driver's seat.

November · Week of _____

REFLECTION

"Look not every man on his own things, but every man on the things of others" (Philippians 2:4).

I want to use this verse to inspire you to become more aware of the next generation—of those that cannot make their own decisions concerning their life. This would include the little girls that are special to you. Is their hair being protected and handled properly, or is their hair an object of inconvenience for the mother and is neglected and put away in braids or disheveled ponytails? Do they still have their edges, or are they broken and thinning already? What about length; do they at least have 12 inches or 2-years-worth of length retention? Take some time to educate the responsible parties for the well-being of the next little girl that may one day be holding this *hairloom*.

RESPONSIBILITY

Mon	
Tues	
Wed	
Thu	
Fri	
Sat	
Sun	

REGIMEN: WEEK 4 TUG-OF-WAR HAIR

This is how I refer to gradual hair loss due to a pulling force applied to the hair. Since the scalp is stable and fixed, the hair cannot contend with the pulling force and has to break because it's not as strong or anchored as the scalp. The strongest, most firmly planted side always wins. This commonly results from frequently wearing hair in a particular tight ponytail, braids, or hair jewelry. The symptoms include mild scalp irritation and swelling in the area of tension that forms tiny bumps or even scabs on the scalp, ultimately resulting in hair breakage. Over time, chronic tension will trigger the skin to go into defense mode and it will form scar tissue (the follicle will close and disallow hair to surface) to prevent further damage to the follicle.

What's the cure? Stop applying tension to the scalp and hair, and it will heal itself.

Hairgistics

Shampoo _____

Conditioner _____

Leave-In _____

Support Product _____

Conditioning time _____

Dryer Time _____ Air dry _____

Protective Style _____

Detangle: Comb _____ Finger _____

Before

Dry	Shedding	Full		
Moist	Breaking	Frizzy		
Oily	Limp	Dull		
Stinky	Heavy	Itchy		
Tangled	Tight	Hard		

After

Dry	Shedding	Full		
Moist	Breaking	Frizzy		
Oily	Limp	Dull		
Stinky	Heavy	Itchy		
Tangled	Tight	Hard		

RELAXATION

Have you ever had a hair and scalp spa day? This is where the environment is set for you to literally lay back on a massage table, place your hair into a shampoo bowl, and relax with music, candles, and a dimly lit ambiance. A skilled professional strategically addresses your scalp and strands while massaging the scalp with just the right amount of pressure. You may want to consider treating yourself to a hair/scalp spa experience before you complete your first successful *hairloom*.

Journemony Time

Dear Loved One,

Challenges create opportunity for you to obtain a different perspective in order
to overcome them. Allow the challenges of life to . . .

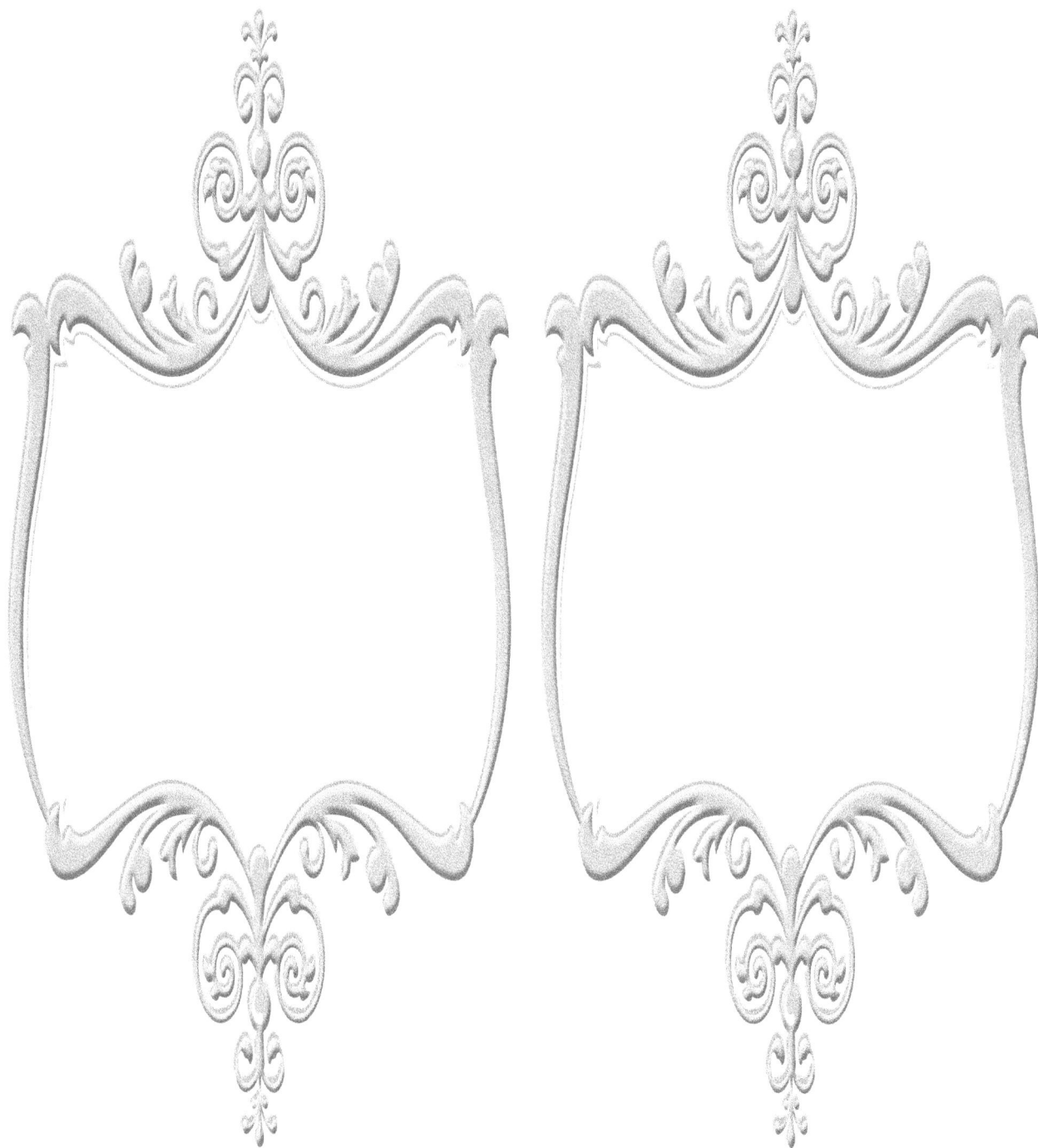

Picture Time

December _____

Season: Cold & Dry

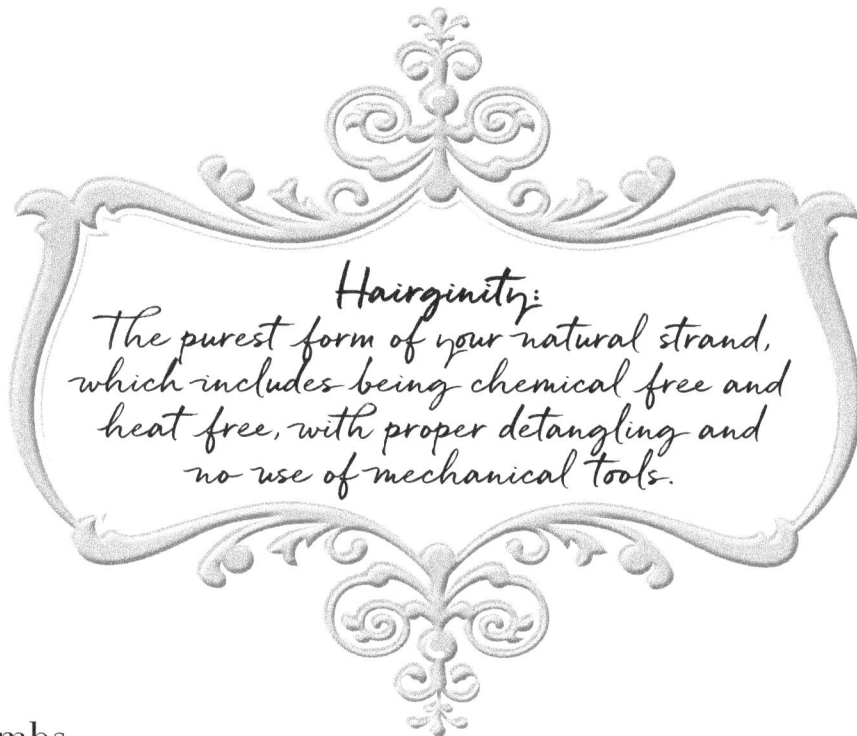

Hairginity:
The purest form of your natural strand,
which includes being chemical free and
heat free, with proper detangling and
no use of mechanical tools.

Hairginity
Week 1: Combs
Week 2: Brushes
Week 3: Bonnets
Week 4: Hair Jewelry

Seasonal Consideration:

Challenge: Keeping the hair and scalp hydrated and covered

Decision: Style choice and hair manipulation

Goal: _____
_____
_____
_____
_____

December · Week of _____

REFLECTION

"Peace, be still" (Mark 4:39).

"Have you ever considered that Jesus, when rebuking the sea, called the storm 'peace'?" (Benjamin Allen Jr.).

What are you going to call the storms and challenges in your life?

_____

_____

Your internal environment will determine how you view your external environment. Take a second look and reconsider what authority you will give to challenges that merely need to be prioritized and appreciated for the life lessons that they bring.

RESPONSIBILITY

Mon	
Tues	
Wed	
Thu	
Fri	
Sat	
Sun	

REGIMEN: WEEK 1 COMBS

Combs are useful for the purpose of parting the hair, removing shedding hair, and smoothing for the purpose of roller setting—and according to research, combs are useful for securing long hair in place, decorating the hair, and matting sections for dreadlocks. For the purpose of this *hairloom*, a part of reclaiming your *hairginity* includes very little to no use of any mechanical tools on the hair, and this includes combs. You may be saying, *You have lost your mind! I need to comb my hair daily.*

However, depending on the style decision, based on the condition of the hair, your hand comb could get the job done just fine. Especially if you are transitioning and have more than one texture and type along the shaft, minimal use of anything other than your hand and an occasional use of the tail of the comb to part the hair will suffice and be safer than using a mechanical comb. A comb should never be used for the purpose of detangling or lifting dandruff or scratching the scalp. You will literally be committing "Hairicide" if you continue these practices. For those that are natural, your hand comb should be your number one go to. Don't knock it till you try it.

Hairgistics

Shampoo _____

Conditioner _____

Leave-In _____

Support Product _____

Conditioning time _____

Dryer Time _____ Air dry _____

Protective Style _____

Detangle: Comb _____ Finger _____

Before

Dry	Shedding	Full		
Moist	Breaking	Frizzy		
Oily	Limp	Dull		
Stinky	Heavy	Itchy		
Tangled	Tight	Hard		

After

Dry	Shedding	Full		
Moist	Breaking	Frizzy		
Oily	Limp	Dull		
Stinky	Heavy	Itchy		
Tangled	Tight	Hard		

RELAXATION

If you started at the beginning of the year, you have learned a lot about yourself by now. I want to commend you for your diligence and commitment to your health and well-being. Relax in the fact that you have not only accomplished much concerning your *hairgistics* but have also experienced 6 inches of new growth. Think of all of the other areas you have experienced growth in as well—some voluntary but others involuntary based on your commitment to take the challenge. Imagine what else you are capable of doing with a little reflection, responsibility, regimen, and relaxation. Now exhale!

December · Week of _____

REFLECTION

Peace is knowing what matters most and making what matters most the focus. What are you focusing on in this season?

_____

_____

I am sure there are many distractions and obligations that could create an environment that robs you of the internal peace that you desire for your life. Take a step back, reevaluate your purpose in everybody's life, and receive the fact that you are not and never will be the source of peace for their lives. You can only maintain your own.

RESPONSIBILITY

Mon	
Tues	
Wed	
Thu	
Fri	
Sat	
Sun	

REGIMEN: WEEK 2 BRUSHES

During this journey, especially if you are in transition, I do not recommend the use of a brush. I know you have heard that brushes stimulate the blood flow, increasing circulation and ultimately supporting hair growth, but guess what . . . without you brushing, your blood is still flowing! And furthermore, you haven't brushed faithfully and consistently every day of your life, and your hair is still growing. Surprise! Therefore, let's not get brand new and start all of these extra practices based on hearsay alone.

You see, what most don't know is that all brushes are not created for the same purpose. Some have bristles that will forcefully detangle, smooth, and flatten the hair into submission with or without support products. This practice not only has the potential to tear or break the hair but also leaves microscopic tears on the scalp as well. Yep, that's why it feels so good to brush with a "good brush," as it is normally called. On the other hand, we have paddle brushes that have the little round balls on the end of each point that are specifically designed for the purpose of smoothing and bringing frizzy hair together. For this journey, a brush will not be needed for the purpose of creating *hairgistics*; therefore, save your money and time.

Hairgistics

Shampoo _____

Conditioner _____

Leave-In _____

Support Product _____

Conditioning time _____

Dryer Time _____ Air dry _____

Protective Style _____

Detangle: Comb _____ Finger _____

Before

Dry	Shedding	Full		
Moist	Breaking	Frizzy		
Oily	Limp	Dull		
Stinky	Heavy	Itchy		
Tangled	Tight	Hard		

After

Dry	Shedding	Full		
Moist	Breaking	Frizzy		
Oily	Limp	Dull		
Stinky	Heavy	Itchy		
Tangled	Tight	Hard		

RELAXATION

Begin to practice relaxing your mind on a daily basis. Determine at the beginning of the day what you will or will not attend to with your thoughts, and obey yourself. No one else can make you think about anything other than what you allow. Remember, we are created to receive and release, and we have free will to voluntarily choose what we meditate or think on.

December · Week of _____

REFLECTION

"Lord, let me do so much good that I don't even remember" (Dr. Christina Rosenthal).

It is important that everything we do for others is free—meaning no obligations or strings attached. Otherwise, we are rewarding a person instead of blessing them. The love we received from Christ came without our work or effort; therefore, we can say that it was a free gift. How many gifts have you given that were really payments or down payments? Let your motive be pure, and give freely, seeking nothing in return.

RESPONSIBILITY

Mon	
Tues	
Wed	
Thu	
Fri	
Sat	
Sun	

REGIMEN: WEEK 3 BONNETS

Bonnets have evolved considerably, and many choices can sometimes make matters more confusing than needed. I recommend protecting the hair any time it will be exposed to external environmental pollutants, at bedtime to protect from the friction and drying effects of the cotton bedding, and when wearing hats in the winter or summer. The only material that should be allowed on the hair is that which does not soak up or dry out the natural oils and support products used for *hairgistics*.

This is why bonnets are normally satin or silk material, to help maintain the moisture level of the hair. Other than material content, we must also consider the shape and how it fits on the head. For the sake of the edges, the bonnet should not rub or cause any friction to the hairline. Therefore, the bonnets that have the elastic bands should be discarded or turned inside out so the satin will have immediate access to the hairline to avoid direct traction and tension. A smooth band that is loosely fitted is recommended, or just a satin pillowcase if you are more of a light sleeper. Also, be sure that the bonnets are clean every time your hair is cleaned, and if this is inconvenient, you may want to purchase more than one.

Hairgistics

Shampoo _____

Conditioner _____

Leave-In _____

Support Product _____

Conditioning time _____

Dryer Time _____ Air dry _____

Protective Style _____

Detangle: Comb _____ Finger _____

Before

Dry	Shedding	Full		
Moist	Breaking	Frizzy		
Oily	Limp	Dull		
Stinky	Heavy	Itchy		
Tangled	Tight	Hard		

After

Dry	Shedding	Full		
Moist	Breaking	Frizzy		
Oily	Limp	Dull		
Stinky	Heavy	Itchy		
Tangled	Tight	Hard		

RELAXATION

Have you ever considered skipping the commercialization of Christmas? This way, you could begin spreading your love language of gifts in January to have more time to give and show your love and appreciation for others throughout the year. This would definitely take the pressure off of this month.

December · Week of _____

REFLECTION

Jesus said, "I am come that they might have life, and that they might have it more abundantly" (John 10:10).

I have heard it said that "Jesus is the reason for the season." May I add that He is the reason that we have the opportunity to have and enjoy life in every season. Do not allow certain seasons to define your ability to enjoy life. Make a decision to create an internal environment of peace that will transcend any season that may present unforeseen challenges or uneventful appeal.

RESPONSIBILITY

Mon	
Tues	
Wed	
Thu	
Fri	
Sat	
Sun	

REGIMEN: WEEK 4 HAIR JEWELRY

Hair jewelry is anything that is applied to the hair other than support products. There are a variety of choices: from clips, to bows, to headbands, to scrunchies, to rubber bands—anything that can be applied to the hair for the purpose of gathering or decorating is considered in this category. What we want to be aware of more than anything is how it feels when it is attached to the hair and scalp. If it bites or pulls or you notice that it has hair in it when you remove it, chuck it! We don't need any fixed apparatus causing unnecessary breakage and tension on the hair that is already in critical condition. It's just not wise. Even rollers should never be worn to bed or laid on in any way.

Hairgistics

Shampoo _____

Conditioner _____

Leave-In _____

Support Product _____

Conditioning time _____

Dryer Time _____ Air dry _____

Protective Style _____

Detangle: Comb _____ Finger _____

Before

Dry	Shedding	Full		
Moist	Breaking	Frizzy		
Oily	Limp	Dull		
Stinky	Heavy	Itchy		
Tangled	Tight	Hard		

After

Dry	Shedding	Full		
Moist	Breaking	Frizzy		
Oily	Limp	Dull		
Stinky	Heavy	Itchy		
Tangled	Tight	Hard		

RELAXATION

Take a deep breath; this month is almost over. If you started this journey at the beginning of the year, hopefully you have taken at least 10 percent of every week to relax and have time for reflection. I would like to believe that you have added at least 10 more years to your life by taking a little time to truly attend to and care for your entire mind, body, and spirit. Balance creates opportunity for health and healing, and you deserve to treat yourself to a life of abundant peace, joy, and love, no matter what your present condition or external environment presents.

Journemony Time

Dear Loved One,

I am so proud of you for . . .

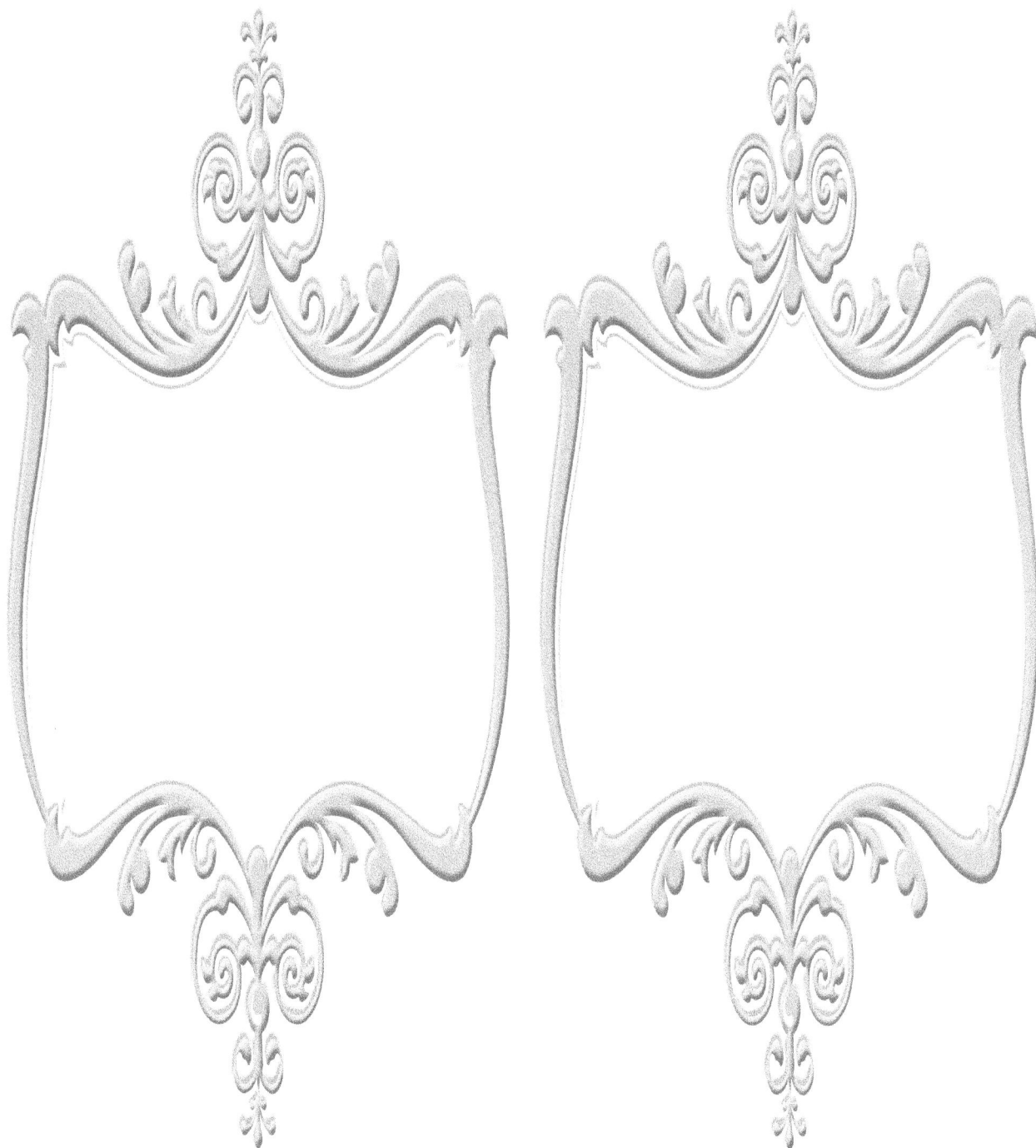

Picture Time

Appendix

The following are the answers to the "Pop Quiz" presented in the introduction:

1. The foundation for a healthy head of hair is to keep the ends trimmed.

    False: *The foundation for a healthy head of hair is balance of internal and external hair/health care needs.*

2. All shampoos serve the same purpose, which is to clean the hair and scalp.

    False: *Moisturizing shampoos do not thoroughly clean the hair and scalp.*

3. Proper conditioning is very important because it helps to repair hair that becomes damaged, thin, and broken.

    False: *Conditioners do not repair the hair; it only conditions the hair to be more manageable.*

4. Brushing can scratch your scalp and tear your hair.

    True: *The use of bristle brushes can scratch your scalp and cause microscopic tears along the shaft of the hair.*

5. The most effective way to remove tangles is by holding the hair at the root and raking through the ends until tangles have been released.

    False: *Finger detangling is the safest and most effective way to loosen tangles.*

6. Shampooing is required when your style does not look presentable.

    False: *Shampooing is required when the hair and scalp are dirty.*

7. The number one cause of hair breakage is using super strength relaxers.

    False: *The number one cause of hair breakage is improper handling and manipulation of the hair.*

8. Dandruff is an indication that hair is growing.

    False: *Dandruff is an indication of an accumulation of dead skin that builds up on the scalp and disperses through the hair.*

9. A sensitive scalp is a damaged scalp.

    True

10. The safest styling technique is a roller set.

    False: *The safest styling technique is reclaiming or maintaining hairginity.*

www.ingramcontent.com/pod-product-compliance
Lightning Source LLC
Chambersburg PA
CBHW081153270326
41930CB00014B/3133